FITNESS FOR THE NEW MILLENNIUM

MARK W. LISKY
WALTER D. ANDZEL PH.D.

ILLUSTRATIONS BY
PETER SHEBELL

KENDALL/HUNT PUBLISHING COMPANY
4050 Westmark Drive   Dubuque, Iowa 52002

Prior to beginning any physical exercise program, it is important that you consult with your physician on how this will impact your individual conditions. The authors highly recommend that you see your physician before starting any fitness program.

This edition has been printed directly from camera-ready copy.

Copyright © 1998 by Mark W. Lisky and Walter D. Andzel

ISBN 0-7872-5237-9

In memory of
Mary Julia Andzel
WDA

To
Dr. Melinda L. Wagner
For awakening the giant within
MWL

FITNESS
FOR THE
NEW
MILLENNIUM

← ——————————————————————— →

Table of Content

Introduction

Fitness may be one of the most confusing activities known to humanity. From fitness facilities across the country, the cry of "there are just so many fitness programs, theories and training styles to choose from, what is a person to do?" can be heard in a great crescendo of frustration. The authors of Fitness for the New Millennium have heard the cry and have decided to take some action to help shed some new light on this confusing but extremely important human activity.

To answer the many perplexing questions of fitness, Fitness for the New Millennium will take a systematic look at the many different aspects of fitness training. This book is designed to take an individual on a step by step process into the art of choosing and building a personal fitness workout program. We'll take a look at some of the facts and theories about fitness exercise. Hopefully at the end, the reader will be able to design a workout program which will specifically match their personal wants, desires, restrictions and lifestyle for the new millennium.

ONE

The Ten Commandments of Fitness Training

Whether you've just started a fitness program for the first time, or you're a veteran fitness fanatic - ironpusher - gym-rat, there are a few training tips that everyone (regardless of level or ability) who trains for fitness should heed. These tips, or "Ten Commandments of Fitness Training", are important because a violation of any one of them may set your fitness goals up like bowling pins, only to be knocked down by an endless circle of frustration. On the other hand, if you use these Commandments as a general guide, they'll keep you heading on a positive course towards the fitness results you want. After all, seeing progressive positive results from your hard fought efforts and sweat is what makes working out exciting, wouldn't you agree?

1) Thou shall not stretch before a proper warm-up

This commandment tops the list for the number one "do not" because it's the one that seems to get violated the most. It's extremely common to see people come out of the locker room and head directly to the mats and start stretching. If you ask them what they're doing, the response is usually "I'm warming up a little before the workout."

Even though their intentions are good and they have the right idea about the need to warm-up prior to exercise, their actions unfortunately are misplaced. In reality, stretching is not a warm-up activity in itself, it is a flexibility activity. The main reason stretching is not used as a warm-up prior to exercise is that stretching is not a heat producing activity. Stretching will not produce energy sufficient to warm-up the body and activate the body's internal systems from a resting state to a workout state.

Also, you should be wary of stretching before a general body warm-up because of the potential situation of muscle trauma and injury caused by stretching cold muscles. Cold muscles are much more receptive to injury than muscles which are properly warmed up.

Stretching is a very important aspect of your total training program and one that should not be overlooked, but make sure it's properly placed in your program. If you're going to stretch make sure it's performed after a general total body warm-up, which leads us to our second Commandment.

2) Thou shall not skip a warm-up prior to strength or fitness training

This is the second most violated rule in exercise training which is seen in every gym, every day. How many times have you seen someone walk into the gym, go directly to a piece of equipment and begin using heavy and maximal weight loads on their second or third set?

If you're in your late teens or early twenties you may be able to get away with this, but it will eventually catch up to you in some form of injury. If you're in your thirties or forties and suffer from chronic and nagging pains in your elbows, shoulders, knees and so on, you may attribute them to the lack of proper warm-up that has accumulated over a period of time.

The importance of general warm-up prior to your exercise program can not be understated and should be mandatory on your program for two basic reasons. The first is that the warm-up period takes the body from a non-active cold state to a ready state of exercise activity. This is necessary because the multi-levels of physiological activities which promote physical progress must be allowed to be "switched on" before they're asked to perform effectively. A mechanic will tell you that immediately driving a car after it's been sitting all night in the winter cold isn't good for the engine and will lessen its life. So it is for the bio-engines that run the human body. This is why in baseball there is something called the bullpen for pitchers to get warmed-up in so they don't go into the game cold and injure their throwing arm.

The other important aspect of warming up is that it gives you a window of opportunity to settle down and mentally prepare on the workout to come. If you've just rushed in from work you may not have time to focus on your workout because your mind is running a thousand miles a minute. The warm-up gives you the time to focus on what you're going to accomplish in the gym that day. This means greater progress from your training time.

So remember to start all your workouts with a general body warm-up. This could be anywhere from fifteen to twenty minutes at a moderate intensity level using any type of aerobic activity, such as a treadmill, step climber, or a stationary bike. Even running in place will do.

3) Thou shall not start a workout with secondary muscle groups prior to a primary muscle group

This Commandment focuses on which exercises go where on a training program in order to keep yourself out of trouble. Through no fault of their own, many individuals tend to start a training session using secondary muscle group exercises, then try to perform primary exercises. The problem here is that the secondary muscle groups tend to support the primary groups. If the secondary muscles are fatigued, they can not support the primary group resulting in an ineffective workout.

An example of this can be found in the triceps and

chest. The triceps being a secondary muscles group, support the motions of the chest during exercises like the bench press. If they're tired because you've worked them to exhaustion prior to training the chest, they cannot properly support the weight loads that the chest can handle.

The major secondary muscle groups which work as a supportive unit with the primary muscle groups are; Shoulders - Triceps for the primary group of the Chest. Biceps which support the primary muscle group of the Back.

4) Thou shall not work the same muscle groups two days in a row

As we saw in Commandment 3, certain muscle groups give support and work as a team with other muscle groups. If you work one of these co-operational groups one day, you should not work another one within the group the following day, because there is no recuperation time period. This violation is seen when someone performs a chest exercises on a Monday, and then decides to work shoulders or triceps on Tuesday, or they work biceps on Wednesday and train back on Thursday. If you're going to train two days in a row, it's better to use a push - pull system where you work your chest, shoulders and triceps one day, and your legs, back and biceps the next.

5) Thou shall not workout at maximum capacity every workout

This is a training Commandment which is violated by almost everyone who works out at one time or another, and is a relic from the old "No Pain No Gain" era. There has been an established belief in fitness that a person will not progress unless a total maximum effort (meaning going to exhaustion) is given every workout. This is completely unfounded.

The body needs time to adapt to the different intensities of training. If every set of every exercise at every workout is taken to failure, there is no recovery or adaptation time given to the body. Without this time to adapt, the body will stagnate. This is why you see so many people in the gym whose strength levels and body shapes have stayed the same for years with no improvement, even though they work out very hard.

There are times when maximal all out efforts are required, but there are many other times when moderate and even submaximal efforts need to be employed in order for the body to recovery and improve. Remember, there are many kinds of training which produce various effects on the human body. High repetitions with low weight, moderate repetitions with moderate weight loads, and low repetitions with high weight loads, all these variations have their place in an exercise program since each one has a different and desirable effect on the body. But whatever kind of training you're doing, you can only perform it at a certain intensity level for a certain time period before you need to change both intensity and types of training.

6) Thou shall not use rest intervals of under 30 seconds if you're using moderate or heavy weights

If you're using heavy weight loads or even moderate weight loads which are close to your maximum lifting abilities, you need to rest more then the traditional 30 seconds before you do another set of the same exercise. The reason for this is that here are many internal bio-systems of the body, both muscular and neuromuscular which work together to help you perform an exercise. Like a car racing at the INDY 500, these systems need a pit stop to refuel. Rest intervals of under 30 seconds when you're using maximal weight loads, simply do not allow enough time for these systems to be refueled and recover before they're asked to perform more work.

What this means in essence, is that you're allowing your body to go back out on the track with a quarter tank of gas while operating at top speed. If you're using moderate to high weight loads, you'll need at least two to three minutes between sets to fully recover and refuel. If that seems like a lot of time to wait in between sets, it is, but it's the way the body works best.

7) Thou shall not walk into the gym without some definite workout plan and program

Be honest with this one. How many times have you gone to the gym and you really didn't know what you were going to do that day? You may have had a general idea of what you wanted to do, like training your legs, but I'm talking about an exact workout plan that keeps you from wandering about the gym lost in indecision. Not having some rudimentary training plan will cost in both wasted training time and inefficient workouts.

A complete workout plan starts with your specific training goals and specific time periods for accomplishing those goals. After this first step is completed, your plan would then include the exercises, sets, reps and weight loads you're going to use every workout within your specified time periods. This step includes what weeks your training intensities levels will be raised and when they will be lowered.

It's obvious that this complete planning takes some thinking about. Your plan must be worked on before you go to the gym, not after you get there, not in the locker room as you change, and not in between sets. If you have some specific training plan, your workouts will be more productive, you'll save time and you'll leave the gym with a new feeling of confidence knowing exactly where you're going in your training, and how you're going to get there.

8) Thou shall not create conflicting workout goals

Violating this Commandment will add unnecessary pressure and unnecessary frustration upon yourself in a world already filled with useless activities. If because of your lifestyle arrangements, time schedule and work schedule, you can only train three times a week for a half an hour or so, use that as the parameters for designing your workout.

Do yourself a favor and stay within realistic boundaries. Do not plan to train five days a week, two hours a day, if you do not have the time. If you do, sooner or later you'll begin to miss workouts, or hurry through workouts in a sloppy manner and the fitness gains you seek will not appear. This will lead to frustration and getting down on yourself, these are two things you do not need in your life.

9) Thou shall not use advanced workouts before you're ready

When we all start on a new endeavor, our enthusiasm sometimes takes priority over our better judgment. This is very common in fitness where you have someone who has been inactive for several years, and decides to take up training. The first day out they tend to do more then they should and they end up with sore and aching muscle for the next week or more. If you're new to exercise or even if you consider yourself an intermediate, give your body time to adapt to a basic workout routine before jumping up to more advanced routines.

Enthusiasm is a great attitude to possess, no doubt, but balance that attitude with patience and good judgment and the rewards will be twice as great.

10) Thou shall not sit on a piece of equipment in between sets

This Commandment is more in the realm of gym etiquette then technical training but can cause just as much frustration as any of the others. If you're resting in between a set of exercises, please don't sit there on a piece of equipment, staring out into space. Move your butt off the piece until you're ready to use it and give somebody else a chance. On the other hand people can't read minds. If you need to use a piece of equipment which somebody is perched on like a bird in a tree, ask them if you can work in with them.

Don't be shy, remember you're a member of the gym just like they are, and who knows, through this simple exchange of courtesy, you may even find the new workout partner you've been looking for.

The Ten Commandments of Fitness

1) Thou shall not stretch before a proper warm-up.
2) Thou shall not skip a warm-up prior to strength or fitness training.
3) Thou shall not start a workout with secondary muscle groups prior to a primary muscle group.
4) Thou shall not work the same muscle groups two days in a row.
5) Thou shall not workout at maximum capacity every workout.
6) Thou shall not use rest intervals of under 30 seconds if you're using moderate or heavy weights.
7) Thou shall not walk into the gym without some definite workout plan and program.
8) Thou shall not create conflicting workout goals.
9) Thou shall not use advanced workouts before you're ready.
10) Thou shall not sit on a piece of equipment in between sets.

TWO

The Seven Basic Building Blocks

Fitness training is individualized and can only be designed according to your particular anatomy, physiological condition and goals. Since no two people have the same body type, height and weight, they stand little chance of attaining the same results if they train identically. So how do you determine which is the best fitness training program for you? The answer lies in understanding the seven basic building blocks of fitness training and evaluating their effects. These basics apply to everyone, but how each one is applied will depend on you.

1. **Universality** - This is defined as the all-around development principle. You must develop strength, cardio and endurance together while training all the major muscles, joints and support structures. Universality will serve as a base for specialized training and development later down the road.

2. **Gradualness** - The physical demands placed on your body must progress gradually in both volume and intensity. Physical ability and your immediate level of fitness will determine your rate of increase. No matter how hard you try, you will not realize significant improvement in a short period of time. The only method known to achieve long-lasting results is to adhere to gradualness. This cannot be over-emphasized. If you reach a plateau in your fitness training, do not become alarmed. It may be an indication that you need to vary your approach.

3. **Progressiveness** - This principle is closely related to gradualness. When stimulating the body to adapt to greater workloads over a period of time, there must be an increase in the amount of intensity used. The increase will be greater when you begin training and

become less when your level of fitness develops

4. **Repetition** - Performing repetitions with high to moderate weight is the only way to learn how to properly perform an exercise and provoke certain physiological changes to take place in your body. When learning how to correctly perform an exercise, performing repetitions will allow you to develop proper technique. If you begin using heavy weights, you will not learn the correct technique. When technique is bad, you will not be working the muscles effectively. This can lead to possible injury.

5. **Consistency** - If you are to realize any change to your appearance, strength, body measurements and body composition you must commit yourself to a regular fitness training schedule. The minimum being two days a week. Your body will respond only when the exercises are performed on a regular basis. This is where you come face to face with your training commitment to achieve your specific fitness goals. Achieving maximum results will require a strong commitment to your workouts and training objectives.

6. **Individualism** - Your health, age, sex, and level of fitness will determine how well you can perform certain exercises and training programs. If you are in your mid-teens, elderly, or in poor fitness, using light weights and performing 8-12 repetitions is advisable. This will allow you to slowly adapt to your weight training program without subjecting yourself to possible injury.

7. **Awareness** - To successfully achieve your weight training goals and objectives, it is necessary to develop an understanding of the basic principles of weight training. With this as the foundation of your training program, it will generate the enthusiasm and desire to make weight training a consistent part of your lifestyle. Knowledge builds muscle and fitness!

It takes not one drop of sweat to put off doing anything

THREE

The Big Four Principles of Progressive Resistance

Fitness training on any level is in actuality an internal balancing act being performed twenty four hours a day, seven days a week. The balance that must be kept is between work (training stress) and recovery. Regardless of what training program or system you're training on, your body will only respond to the correct balance between these two integrated factors.

Stress the body, let it adapt and recover from that stress, and then stress it again. Repeat this cycle with the correct ratio between rest and recovery and the body will respond by changing its appearance. Repeat this cycle with the incorrect ratio, and the body will respond with the mother of all negative side effects, overtraining. In order to help determine the correct work / recovery ratio, you must familiarize yourselves with the "Big Four" principles of fitness.

The first principle is the "**Overload**." Simply stated, this principle means that stress (in this case increases in training intensity) should be added in a controlled and progressive pattern only after the body has had time to adapt. In order for the body to fully adapt, the same training loads need to be repeated for the duration of one cycle of training. This cycle is measured in total number of workouts performed. Anywhere from two to three workouts using the same training methods and intensities will constitute one cycle.

This means if you're training with weights for your chest, shoulders and triceps in one workout which is repeated two or three times a week, you need to use the same loads, sets and reps for the entire weekly cycle in order to adapt. The reasoning behind this is that the first workout of the week stresses the body, the second two workouts adapt the body to the stress. The following week, work intensities can safely be increased, creating a new cycle.

The problem with many people is that they change the training intensities workout to workout. They go light one day, the next workout go intense and so on. This pattern locks the body in a perpetual guessing game. Because of this, adaptation and recovery from the stress never takes place. This will only last so long before chronic fatigue symptoms and overtraining begin to appear. The next aspect of the Overload is that you need to string several of these weekly cycles together to form a chain.

Picture it like a flight of ascending stairs, with the intensity levels slightly increasing week to week. This controlled progression will provide constant, long term training gains throughout the year. Note that on every third or fourth week, you'll need to include one cycle of reduced training intensity. This week, which is often referred to as a "down-loading" week, will add to your recovery process.

The second principle is "**Overcompensation.**" Overcompensation is the sister to Overload and actually takes place between individual workouts. During, and immediately after a workout, the body's internal systems are thrown out of balance. During these times various kinds of fatigue set in. Nutrient fatigue, muscular fatigue, neuromuscular fatigue and so on. When fatigue sets in, the body tries desperately to get back into balance. If there is the proper amount of sleep, the proper amount of time before another workout is performed, and the proper amount of nutrients, the body not only comes back into balance, but actually overcompensates and slightly improves. This overcompensation is where the improvement in physical appearance takes place.

Put enough of these overcompensation cycles together and the body will continually improve. The flip side of this equation is that if there is not enough recovery between workouts to counter the effects of fatigue, then overcompensation cannot take place. Not only will you fail to reach a positive balance, but the body will slightly undercompensate. String enough of these undercompensation cycles together and normal fatigue will become chronic, leaving you drained of training energy.

The third principle is "**Rest-Intervals.**" The basis of this principle is simple. As the weight loads increase, the rest intervals (RI) must also increase in direct proportion. The reason for this is both biochemical and neuromuscular. Remember that when you perform work, such as lifting weights, your body uses various fuels to give you energy.

At low and moderate intensities (approximately 50% to 70% of maximal loads), your body basically uses two fuels, adenosine triphosphate (ATP) and creatine triphosphate (CP). Depletion of these fuels occur rapidly as you perform your set. It may take up to three minutes to allow these fuels to be fully restored. If your RI is only thirty seconds, approximately fifty percent of ATP/CP is restored. If this is the case, then even before your workout is completed, the process of undercompensation has begun. At maximal intensities (approximately 85% to 100% maximal loads), the neuromuscular system plays an important role in the lifting of maximal weight loads. At these heavy loads, not only must the fuel systems be restored, but the firing impulses of the nerves must also be restored.

This may take up to five minutes. If you use short RI while using maximal loads, the nerve impulses which tell the muscle to contract are greatly effected by fatigue and may not fire with the proper degree of force, speed or frequency. This situation, if allowed to continue, will also trigger the onset of overtraining

The last principle is the "**Weight Load Pattern**". In progressive weight training for fitness, there are two major weight load ranges, maximal and submaximal. These ranges are based on percentages of an individual's maximum strength levels. Maximal weight loads are those loads between 85% and 100% of an individual's maximum strength levels. These percentages of weight loads are used for increasing strength levels and increasing muscle density. The rep ranges when training with maximal loads may be from 1 to 6 reps per set for 2 to 4 sets.

Submaximal weight loads have two ranges. These ranges are between 50% to 85% of a person's maximum strength levels. The first range is from 70% to 85%. This weight load range is best used to produce increases in muscle size. The rep ranges may be from 6 to 10 reps, depending upon the load. Anywhere from 4 to 5 sets may be used.

The next range of submaximal weight loads fall between 50% to 70% of maximal strength levels. This range of weight loads is generally used to prepare the body, especially the joints, for the physical demand of higher loads. This range may also be used after a layoff period or injury to help the body get back into action. It also may be used very effectively between cycles of maximal load workouts to allow the body to recovery. The reps ranges here may be between 10 to 15 for a total of 5 to 6 sets.

Overload

Overcompensation

Rest-Intervals

𝔚𝔢𝔦𝔤𝔥𝔱 𝔏𝔬𝔞𝔡 𝔓𝔞𝔱𝔱𝔢𝔯𝔫

FOUR

No Pain
No Gain?
NO WAY!

One of the greatest cliches of the fitness movement is that in order to get a fit, athletic body you have to pay an awful price in physical pain. While there is disagreement over just how much pain or discomfort is beneficial during a workout, one concept seems clear and is universally agreed upon; there is "good pain" and "bad pain".

The good pain is synonymous with the "burn". Indeed this may be described as a mild burning sensation in the muscles you're working on or in your lungs when you are doing an aerobic workout. The muscle burn is caused by lactic acid that quickly dissipates after your workout. The "good" pain can also be a heavy feeling in your muscles after a long strenuous workout, signaling fatigue.

The bad pain usually appears suddenly and sharply, sometimes with a snap or a pull. If you feel a pain in a joint, that's bad pain. Also sharp, piercing pains in your neck and chest are definitely something to be concerned with. Likewise, if the minor aches you experience when you start a workout go away, that is probably not "bad" pain, but if it persists or worsens, it is. In general, persistent pain can indicate muscle pulls, tendonitis, or stress fractures, all of which can occur from doing too much too soon.

For beginners it is sometimes difficult to tell the difference between good and bad pain and even seasoned athletes often ignore the warning signs of injury. Bur experiences should teach you how to differentiate between the two. It should be clear as the difference between night and day.

Without experiencing some degree of good pain during a workout, you are not likely to be making progress in your training program. This is because positive training involves progressive overload which stresses the body past what it's used to, which forces it to adapt to a new level and thus increase its functional capacity. Without overload there is no adaptation.

How much of a good pain is a good thing depends on your training goals. When a person moves from training recreational to competitive training, they have to stress the body intensely. In terms of training for health you never have to hurt or be uncomfortable. The key to differentiating between bad and good pain is that you have to know your own body along with guidance from sensitive personal trainers, coaches or sports medicine practitioners. This may be the best way any person has to monitor just how much pain will promote improvement rather than damage. Table 1 gives guidelines for a hard sensible workout. Remember pain in and of itself is not the objective. Understanding it and learning to deal with its idiosyncrasies can teach you many lessons, not the least of which is the secret of how to adopt a balanced view towards training and your life.

TABLE 1
Avoiding "Bad" Pain

• Pay attention to danger signs such as muscular cramps and a persistent headache
• Use good equipment, always insist on a proper fit
• Reduce tension - utilize techniques such as massage, whirlpools, biofeedback, and deep breathing
• Maintain your strength-training muscles in balanced pairs
• Warm up - (10 -15 minutes)

FIVE

Muscle Composition

Before we can develop specific fitness training programs, we need to take a brief look at the human machine. As an individual it is important for you to have a basic knowledge of how the body works. A look into how the human machine functions is necessary if many of the aspects of fitness training are going to be understood. It is like owning a car, you do not have to be a mechanic to drive, but some basic understanding of proper care and maintenance of the engine is needed to keep it in good running condition

The first system of the body we will look at is skeletal muscle which is responsible for all movement. Without muscles, we certainly could not function. Skeletal muscle tissue is attached to our bones and when it contracts our muscles move.

A skeletal muscle is composed of hundreds, thousands of tens of thousands of skeletal muscle fibers depending on the muscle's size. Muscle fibers are highly specialized to produce tension and movement. They are cylindrical with a diameter significantly smaller than a human hair which are barely visible to your eye without an electron microscope. The thickness or diameter of a fiber is essential in determining the strength producing capacity of the fiber. Muscle fiber length is highly variable between muscles. This is determined by genetics and muscle location (ex thighs vs. calves).

The structure that surrounds a single muscle fiber and keeps all of its contents within is called the basement membrane. This basement membrane plays an important role in injury repair. The post exercise pain that you might feel a day or two after a hard workout could be the result of microscopic tears in the basement membrane of several muscle fibers. After you workout the first repairs that are made are to lay down a new scaffolding that replaces an injured basal membrane. Remember a muscle will not grow or get stronger unless this membrane is intact.

Several types of connective tissue maintain the integrity of the muscle. The endomysium is a membrane that covers the outside of each muscle fiber and covers the basement membrane. It prevents fibers from stretching too far. The perimysium is the next membrane. It binds 100-150 muscle fibers into groups called bundles or fascicule. These bundles are held together by the epimysium or fascia which is literally the top of the muscle. The epimysium connects muscles to tendons which attach muscle to bone.

The largest functional unit in a muscle is called a myofibril. There are thousands of them lying side by side in a single muscle fiber. A muscle fiber grows as a result of weight training by an increase in the number of myofibrils. As a result of these new myofibrils the fiber diameter and its cross sectional area increases. These increases in muscle fiber size will increase the growth of the entire muscle.

Myofibrils can be subdivided into box like units known as sacromeres. Sacromeres are arranged end to end with an average length of 2 - 2.5 microns or two thousands of a millimeter. Muscles with very long fibers have more sacromeres end to end than muscles that have short muscle fibers. The number of sacromeres in a fiber can increase and this is dependent upon whether the muscle is trained with resistance.

Although sarcomere are the force generating units, smaller thick and thin filaments called myofilaments, are the main constituents of the sacromeres. Thick (myosin) and thin (actin) filaments lay side by side in sacromeres. This gives a regular pattern of dark and light bands or a striated appearance to the muscle fiber. Skeletal muscle is the only striated tissue we have. A closer look at these myofilaments shows paddle like rods (cross bridges) on the thick filaments. The thin filaments appear like a twisted pearl necklace.

It has been hypothesized that the cross bridges of the myosin filament attach to the thin filament during contraction and pull on the thin filament. Specifically when the brain initiates a series of electrical signals that stimulate a release of calcium inside the muscle fibers. This permits the myosin cross bridge to move and attach to actin. The cross bridge swings out and attaches to stimulated sites on the actin and pulls on the actin.

Because the thin filaments are anchored to the end of the sarcomere at a Z line, each half of the sarcomere moves towards the center. This occurs because the thick filament pulls on the thin filament and does not move itself thus causing the sarcomere to shorten. When enough sacromeres in fibers shorten, the entire muscle will shorten and bones will move.

An interesting characteristic of filaments is that the filament does not change in its protein content with weight training but the number of thin filaments will increase or decrease with training or detraining. In contrast, the thick filament especially the cross bridges change with weight training.These changes effect the thickness of a muscle fiber and thus the size.

It is generally agreed that three individual human skeleton muscle fibers exist: Two subtypes of fast fibers-identified as type 11b and 11a, and a slow fiber identified as type 1. However, recent evidence has identified the existence of two new skeletal muscle fibers in rats: Type 11d- identified as a fast fiber and type 1a- identified as a slow fiber.

Though some muscle groups are known to be composed of predominantly fast or slow fibers, most muscle groups in the body contain an equal mixture of both slow and fast fiber types. The percentages of the respective fiber types contained in skeletal muscles can be influenced by genetics, blood levels and hormones and the weight training techniques or methods used by an individual. Type 11b and type 11a have a large anaerobic capacity and are most influenced by weight training. For example, weight training results in a reduction of the percent of the type 11b fibers and an increase in the percent of type 11a fibers. Table 1 shows the typical composition of fibers of elite athletes and non athletes.

TABLE 1		
Muscle Fiber Composition in Elite Athletes and Non Athletes		
Sport	Type 1 Slow /	Type 11b & 11a Fast
Distance Runners	70% - 80%	30% - 20%
Track Sprinters	25% - 30%	75% - 70%
Weight Lifters	45% - 55%	55% - 45%
Non Athletes	47% - 53%	53% - 47%

Muscles increase in strength and size by being forced to contract at tensions near their maximums. If muscles are not overloaded then there is no improvement in strength. Today, the perfect weight training regimen remains controversial. There does not appear to be a magic formula for strength training that meets the needs of all of us. Don't be surprised by this conclusion given the fact that all of us vary in our responses to training loads due to differences in fitness levels. Therefore the exercise prescription must be tailored for each individual.

Free Weight versus Machines

Over the past several years, much controversy has centered around the question of whether training with free weights, barbells and dumbbells, produces greater strength gains. Recent studies argue that strength training using free weights is superior to training with many commercial weight machines for the following reasons:

1. Free weights provide movement versatility.
2. They allow a greater specificity of training than weight machines.
3. Training with free weights involves large muscle mass and multi segment exercises, which force an individual to control both balance and body stability.

In conclusion, while we do not have the choice of selecting our genes, we can carefully choose the manner in which we train to get the most adaptive changes within the muscles. This is the only way to optimize our God given genetic potential. Although genetics help us greatly, hard work and proper training have a lot to say about who is successful and those who only wish they were!

"An interesting characteristic of filaments is that the filament does not change in its protein content with weight training but the number of thin filaments will increase or decrease with training or detraining"

SIX

Overtraining
The Kiss
of Death

Overtraining is often referred to as the "kiss of death" to the serious athlete. Unfortunately, exercise science is only taking the first baby steps to understand overtraining. The research literature on overtraining is largely descriptive and very little information on dose response relationships. The experimental information has been contradictory and suffers from problems of definition. Few agree on what overtraining is. Moreover, and not insignificantly, the discovery of one or more markers of overtraining is possibly the "holy grail" of exercise science. So what is overtraining, what are the signs and how does one avoid it?

There are two types of overtraining, general and local. General overtraining affects the whole body producing stagnation and decreases physical performance. When local training occurs, only one specific body part of muscle group is affected. Local overtraining can be experienced by most persons involved in weight training and is recognized by soreness and stiffness after performing a particular exercise.

When overtraining is not acknowledged and allowed to become serious, it can take weeks, or even months for your body to recover. Overtraining must not be confused with exhaustion. Exhaustion is a reaction to the short term imbalance between stress and how your body is adapting to it. Overtraining is the result of a prolonged imbalance with many characteristics. It is important to understand and recognize the warning signs of overtraining and take the necessary steps to alleviate the problem before it gets worse.

The following symptoms can be used to identify

an approaching "overtrained" condition.

1. You experience a noticeable decrease in strength of performance level.
2. Overall fatigue. You don't recover from previous workouts as well as you did before. You become susceptible to headaches, colds and fever blisters.
3. General muscle soreness. You experience a slow, general increase in muscle soreness and stiffness after a workout.
4. You sleep longer than normal and still feel tired.
5. You begin to realize a drop in body weight. This is an easy sign to spot when no effort is being made to lose weight.
6. Your resting heart rate is higher than normal. To check your resting heart rate take your pulse everyday under the same conditions. If your resting heart rate is ten beats higher than normal, your metabolism has not recovered from the previous workout. It normally takes 90 minutes to 2 hours to return to normal, even after a short work out.
7. Your coordination has become impaired. It has become difficult to perform exercises with the same pace and coordination you had in previous workouts.
8. Your body temperature is higher than normal. You begin to feel hot and feverish. This is an important sign that you may be reaching the point of heat exhaustion or heat stroke.
9. You begin to lose your appetite. This could be one of the reasons for a decrease in body weight.
10. The recovery time between sets and workouts is longer than normal.

11. You experience a swelling of the lymph nodes in your neck, groin, or armpits. This, along with an increased body temperature is a symptom requiring immediate attention.

12. You become psychologically and emotionally drained. This includes increased nervousness, depression, inability to relax or poor motivation.

In order to avoid overtraining simply change exercises, training volume, training intensity, training frequency, training duration or any combination of these. Although you should use this idea sparingly, it should be built into your training program. Building in stage of phase-like alterations in your training is referred to as "cycle" training or "periodization".

The simplest, most practical, and most effective method for avoiding overtraining is rest. This does not mean bed rest, but merely a reduction in training demands. Although this seems obvious, you probably already know how seductive rest-avoidance is to you. Remember your body has a limited capacity to adapt in a short period of time and when it is over stressed, you will begin to experience some or all the symptoms of overtraining.

"Overtraining is the result of a prolonged imbalance with many characteristics. It is important to understand and recognize the warning signs of overtraining and take the necessary steps to alleviate the problem before it gets worse"

REVIEW QUESTIONS

A. List 5 of the Ten Commandments of fitness and briefly explain their importance.

_____

_____

_____

_____

_____

_____

_____

_____

_____

_____

_____

_____

_____

B. List the Seven Building Blocks of Fitness Training.

1._____   5._____
2._____   6._____
3._____   7._____
4._____

C. Explain OverCompensation

_____

_____

_____

_____

_____

_____

_____

_____

_____

_____

_____

D. Briefly describe the composition of a skeletal muscle.

_____
_____
_____
_____
_____
_____
_____
_____
_____
_____
_____
_____
_____
_____
_____
_____
_____

E. List the warning signs of overtraining.

_____
_____
_____
_____
_____
_____
_____
_____
_____
_____
_____
_____
_____
_____
_____

SEVEN

Warming-Up The Key to Fitness Success

It's unfortunate that many people tend to brush off performing a proper warm-up prior to a training session. "I don't have enough time to warm-up and workout too," usually leads the list of avoidance excuses. But when all is said and done, skipping a warm-up weakens the foundation of any fitness training program. In order to capitalize on the benefits provided by warming-up, it's important to understand that the warm-up period is not a separate entity from the exercise program itself. It should be regarded as an integral part of the whole process of workout conditioning.

Basically, the warm-up period takes the body from a cold non-active state, to an "on guard" ready state for action. This change from non-active to active is accomplished by increasing body temperature through some form of aerobic activity. When this occurs, the benefits, both physiological and psychologically are many.

Physiologically, increasing body temperature prior to working out decreases the environmental factors which cause muscle and joint injuries. This is especially relative to injuries which stem from performing static or ballistic stretching prior to a complete warm-up. It has also been shown that warming-up may increase the speed in which muscles contract and relax, allowing for less viscous resistance and greater muscular efficiency.

Another interesting fact is that warming-up allows for greater oxygen utilization by the muscles. This situation occurs because blood releases oxygen more easily at higher temperatures. Finally, a proper warm-up may help to increase the efficiency of the neuromuscular system by allowing a more productive nerve transmission to the muscles. This is an important aspect when you're training with heavy weight loads, and it's why a person may be up to twenty percent stronger in a complete warmed up state.

Psychologically, the warm-up plays a major role in preparing the mind to focus on the tasks which lay ahead. This "window of opportunity" for focusing the mind is another very important aspect to physical training. An aspect which stems from controlling the internal dialog which goes on in our minds every waking minute. When we walk into a gym to train, sometimes our minds can be going about a mile a minute. We think about the fight we had with our spouse, or the project for work that must be completed.

These random thoughts must be gathered and controlled if we are going to have a serious workout. Therefore, like a magnifying glass collect light to a focus point which can ignite a fire, the warm-up period allows us a time to collect our wandering thoughts to a single focus point. A point which can ignite an inner fire, whereby we increase workout productivity tenfold.

Generally, the warm-up period is broken into two separate phases. First, the "general warm-up" phase is performed. This could be any aerobic activity which raises body temperature. Remember, we're trying to increase body temperature, not exhaust the body. Sixty minutes of high impact aerobics which leaves your tongue dragging on the floor is a workout, not a warm-up.

In the general warm-up, a good sign that its effects are kicking in is when you start to break out into a sweat. Obviously, the environmental temperature of the gym will play a role in sweating. A good rule of thumb is that the general warm-up should be between fifteen and twenty-five minutes at a moderate intensity level. Again, any moderate activity will do. Calisthenics, running, skipping rope, bike riding, playing basketball or even shadow boxing, all could be used as a general warm-up.

Try to vary the general warm-up phases as much as possible. One workout, shoot some hoops. The next workout ride the bike, and the next shadowbox. Adding variety will keep boredom away and will introduce a crosstraining element into your workouts.

The second phase of the warm-up period which is extremely important in weight training is the "specific warm-up". Here you will be performing the exact exercises from your main weight training workout, except you'll be using very light weight loads. The best procedure to use in the specific warm-up is to perform one or two sets of all your exercises in a circuit manner (moving from one to another). Give yourself about a thirty second rest interval between exercises.

For the specific warm-up, use about thirty to thirty-five percent of your maximal weight load capacity for twenty or more repetitions. These light loads will allow your neuromuscular system to begin anticipating the exact exercise movement that you'll be using in your main workout. Using these light weight loads will also help reduce the potential for injury when you begin using heavier loads. Once you have completed your circuit of exercises, take a few minutes and begin the main part of your training. Your complete warm-up period is now over.

Now that you understand the need for including a complete warm-up period as part of your weight training program. You may want to leave for the gym a little bit earlier. Remember, not only will your training gains come quicker, but you'll be stronger, you ability to focus will increase and your chances of injuries will decrease. It may take some getting use to, but give it a try for a few weeks.

Instead of making excuses not to warm-up, find a way to make the time!

EIGHT

Stretching The Inside Story

In the sixties and seventies, the typical battle cry against fitness training with weights was, "if you lift a weight you'll become so muscle bound that you won't be able to touch your toes or raise your arms above your head."

In some ways this view was correct though taken out of content (the point being that 95% of average people who don't weight train can't touch their toes either). Traditional progressive weight training for fitness without doing supplemental stretching may cause some loss of flexibility.

Losing flexibility isn't a necessary outcome of training, it's a freely chosen situation. People involved in fitness for the most part simply do not stretch. Throwing all technical reasons aside, the reason many people don't stretch is because stretching is time consuming and they feel it will not change appearance of the body. So on the surface, the question is why should someone waste valuable training time stretching?

The answer is simply that flexibility is an important function of the human body, without which the movements of the bodily segments can be restricted. Also, stretching increases the range of motion of muscles and joints thereby allowing a greater range of development. Increasing your flexibility can also have a great impact on reducing physical injuries.

The two major stretching methods used today are *static stretching* and *controlled ballistic* stretching. Static stretching is when you reach your limit of a certain stretch and you hold that for a count of ten or more seconds. You then relax and repeat the stretch. Controlled ballistic stretching is performed by using a controlled bounce motion the end of the stretch, usually ten bounces to a stretch for three sets. Ballistic stretching was labeled dangerous by many experts. This label is uncalled for and stemmed from misunderstanding this dynamic form of stretching. Ballistic stretching is perfectly safe, but only when the body is completely warmed up.

Stretching Criteria

A. Use in the warm up portion of a workout after raising the body's temperature.
B. Use for maintaining normal range of motion.
C. Use in the cool down portion of the work out.

General Rules

Do:

a. Stretch slowly, remain in control of movement.
b. Hold the stretch, work up to about 60 seconds.
c. Feel the stretch in the belly (center) of the muscle. If there is pain in the joint or muscle tremors, STOP!!
d. Stop if "ouch" pain is felt.
e. Warm up muscles before stretching.
f. Breathe normally.
g. Stretch after activities.

Do Not:

a. Lock a joint or hyperextend a joint. (Bend pat the neutral position)
c. Arch the low back or neck.
   Forceful or weight bearing arching should not be done.
d. Perform fast exercise or swinging movement.

This develops momentum and reduces muscle action.

e. Over bend a joint.

f. Hold your breath.

AVOID THE FOLLOWING:

1. Head Rolls
2. Shoulder Stand Plow Bicycle
3. Arm Circles
4. Waist Circles
5. Back Bends
6. Prone Arch
7. Straight Leg Sit ups or with feet held down
8. Leg Lifts
9. Straight Leg Toe Touch
10. Hurdler's stretch
11. Deep Knee Bends or Squats
12. Splits

Stretch Out Program		
Stretch	Sets	Time
1. Neck Stretch		
Left Right Center	2-3	30 seconds
2. Shoulder Stretch	2-3	
3. Standing		
Thigh Stretch	2-3	20-30 seconds
4. Calf Stretch Straight	1-2	30 seconds
5. Seated Groin Stretch	2-3	30 seconds
6. Straight Body Stretch	2-3	
7. Low Back Cat Stretch	2-3	30 seconds
8.Seated Hurdlers Stretch	2	30 seconds
9. Knee Pulls	2	30 seconds

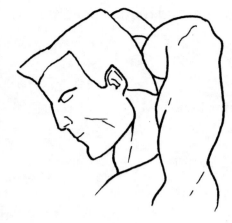

Neck Stretch Forward

To perform this stretch simply place both hands behind the neck and slowly stretch the head forward

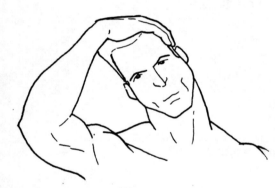

Neck Stretch Side

To perform this stretch place one hand on the side of the head and slowly stretch the head toward the shoulder. Repeat on opposite side

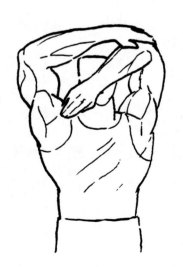

Shoulder Stretch

To perform this stretch place one arm behind your head with the elbow pointing up. Hold the raised elbow and slowly stretch it towards the head. Repeat on opposite side

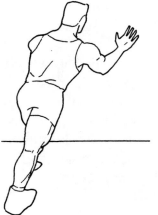

Standing Calf Stretch

To perform this stretch face a wall in a lunge position with both hands against the wall for support. Raise up on the toes of the rear leg and slowly stretch the calf. Repeat on opposite side.

Standing Thigh Stretch

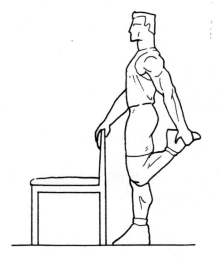

To perform this stretch hold a chair for support as you raise your foot up behind you. Grasp the foot with your hand and slowly pull the foot up towards you're rear. Repeat on opposite side.

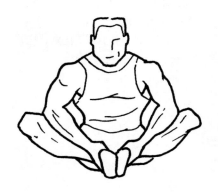

Seated Groin Stretch
To perform this stretch sit on the floor with your legs straddled and your feet together. Slowly push your knees towards the floor as you hold your feet.

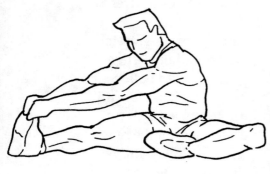

Seated Inside Hurdler Stretch

To perform this stretch sit on the floor with one leg straddled straight and the other bent in. Slowly stretch towards your straight leg. Repeat on other side.

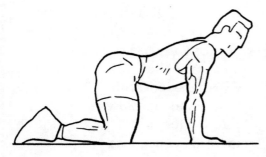

Low Back Cat Stretch

To perform this stretch place both hands and knees on the floor with your back straight or slightly arched. Slowly stretch your lower back by rounding it up. Hold and slowly lower back to the starting position and repeat.

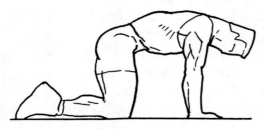

Straight Body Stretch

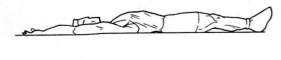

To perform this stretch lay on the floor with arms straight over your head legs straight. Slowly stretch your legs down and your arms up.

Single Leg Knee Pull

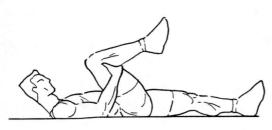

To perform this stretch lay on the floor with one leg bent and the other leg straight. Hold the back of the bent knee and slowly pull the knee up. Repeat on other side

Double Leg Knee Pull

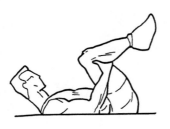

To perform this stretch lay on the floor with both legs bent. Hold the back of both knees and slowly pull the knees up.

NINE

AEROBICS
Overview

An essential part of your overall fitness program should be aerobic training. You should be performing aerobic activities throughout the year. The purpose of aerobic work are for warm up, enhancing recovery, weight control and to build an aerobic base to enhance sports training. Also, performing moderate aerobic activity will assist your body in replenishing fuel to the muscles and remove waste products.

Activities which develop increased oxygen transportation and utilization are referred to as "aerobic exercises". The word aerobic itself means "with oxygen" and indicates that the energy produced to do the work utilizes an oxygen (O_2) system. By increasing the capacity of our aerobic system, you can have a much more efficient body.

Also, aerobic training produces positive training effects on many other systems of the body such as the circulatory, respiratory, muscular and endocrine. Through aerobic training the body increases its capacity to bring in oxygen and transport the oxygen to the necessary areas of the body and then can use the O_2 to produce energy. Examples of aerobic training are aerobic dance (low impact, step aerobics, etc.) bicycling, treadmill, jogging, rollerblading and steppers.

Aerobic training follows the same overload principle which is used in strength training and conditioning. This entails subjecting the cardiovascular systems to loads greater than those to which they are accustomed. The overload causes the system to adapt and increase its total capacity to perform more physical work.

```
┌─────────────────────────────────────────────┐
│                  TABLE 1.                     │
│     Overload Variables for Aerobic Training   │
│                                               │
│ Intensity:    How Hard                        │
│ Increase the rate of speed                    │
│ Increase the slope (treadmill)                │
│ Increase the resistance (bike)                │
│                                               │
│ Duration:    How Long                         │
│ Increase the time                             │
│ Increase the distance                         │
│                                               │
│ Frequency:   How Often                        │
│ Increase the number of workouts               │
└─────────────────────────────────────────────┘
```

TABLE 1.
Overload Variables for Aerobic Training

Intensity: How Hard
Increase the rate of speed
Increase the slope (treadmill)
Increase the resistance (bike)

Duration: How Long
Increase the time
Increase the distance

Frequency: How Often
Increase the number of workouts

As with strength training there are training variables in an aerobic training program to control the overload. These being intensity, duration, frequency and mode of activity. Table 1. Shows various components of these variables.

It must be noted here that specific body systems require specific overloads, therefore an overload for cardio-respiratory systems are different from that necessary to bring about strength gains or flexibility changes.

An athletes aerobic training program should elicit an intensity of 60% to 90% of their maximum heart rate (MHR), this is referred to as the "exercise benefit zone" (EBZ). Aerobic training that causes the heart rate (HR) to increase to the low end of the EBZ will cause skeletal muscles to use fatty acids as a source of energy. Fifteen to sixty minutes of aerobic training is the ideal range of duration for an athlete.

Duration is dependent on the intensity of the activity. In order to burn fat, lower intensity activities should be conducted over a longer period of time. Because of the importance of the "total athlete fitness" effect and the fact that it's more readily attained in a longer duration programs, and because the potential of injury is associated with high intensity aerobic activities, lower to moderate training of longer duration is recommended.

The frequency of aerobic training should be from three to five days per week. Table 2. Shows the minimum overload prescription for improving aerobic athletic fitness, and Table 3. Shows the recommendation for improving athletic fitness and lowering body fat.

TABLE 2.
Minimum Progressive Overload for Aerobic Training

Intensity = 60%-90% of Maximum Heart Rate (per min)
Duration = 15 minutes in EBZ
Frequency = 3 times per week- progress to 5 times

TABLE 3.
Progressive Overload For Body Fat Loss

Intensity = Exercise at low end of EBZ
Duration = 30-60 min
Frequency = 3 times per week- progress to 5 times

A fairly valid and reliable indicator of intensity can be obtained by measuring the HR obtained during participation in aerobic training. In order to determine the recommended HR to achieve a training effect, you must know your MHR. To determine your HR you must be able to count your pulse, this can be most easily done by placing the middle fingers over the carotid artery alongside the esophagus in the neck or over the radial artery on the thumb side of the wrist (see Figure 1).

If you use the carotid artery do not use too much

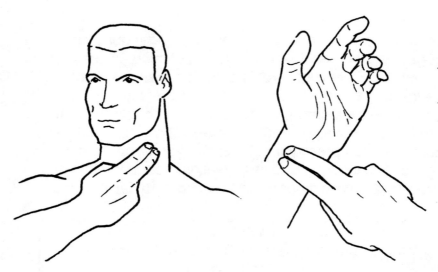

Figure 1

pressure, excessive pressure while taking a pulse may cause the heart rate to slow down by a reflex action. After you have determined your heart rate, start counting with the first count of zero. To directly determine your MHR you could measure the pulse after an all out endurance run or walk. This type of testing is NOT REC-OMMENDED unless approved by your personal physician.

Another easier and safer technique is to approximate your MHR by subtracting your age from 220. For example, an athlete twenty years of age would have an estimated maximal heart rate of two hundred beats per minute (220- 20 = 200). The HR necessary to bring out a training effect is between 60% and 90% of your MHR. To determine the rate you must achieve to ensure aerobic training is a very simple matter. Take 60% of your MHR to find the lowest pulse you should have while training, and 90% of your MHR to estimate the highest pulse rate during an aerobic training session.

Table 4. Shows the computational procedure for determining your EBZ and Table 5. contains the average maximal heart rates and target zones for training effects for selected age groups. If your age is not listed, compute the EBZ as previously explained. It's important that to count the pulse immediately upon stopping the aerobic exercise to determine HR because it does begin to decrease quite rapidly once the exercise is slowed or stopped. Try to find your pulse within five seconds and count the number of beats for ten seconds, then multiply by six to determine your estimated HR for one minute.

A twelve week aerobic program has been set up using the principles of periodization. This program consists of the overload variables, it starts with an intensity of 60% max HR for 15 minutes duration which are the minimal starting recommendation. For the first two weeks the overload is increased and in the third week the overload is decreased (recovery).

1. Rest in bed or sit in a chair.
2. Place the index and forefinger at the base of the thumb side of your opposite wrist (see illustration). Do not use your thumb here.
3. Lightly press your fingers into your arm and you should feel your constant pulse.
4. Count the number of beats that you feel in fifteen seconds.
5. Multiply the number by four and you have your resting heart rate per minute.

TABLE 4.
Computing Your EBZ In Predicted maximum HRM = 220 - your age

Your Predicted maximum HRM_____
Minimum EBZ = Predicted Max HRM x 60%
Your minimum EBZ = _____
Maximum EBZ = Predicted Max HRM x 90%
Your Maximum EBZ_____

TABLE 5.
Average Maximal Heart Rates
and Target Training Zones

AGE	MHR	60%	65%	70%	75%	80%	85%	90%
10	210	126	136	147	158	168	179	189
15	205	123	133	144	154	164	174	185
20	200	120	130	140	150	160	170	180
25	195	117	127	137	146	156	166	176
30	190	114	123	133	143	152	162	171
35	185	111	120	130	139	148	157	167
40	180	108	117	126	135	144	153	162
45	175	105	114	123	131	140	149	158
50	170	102	110	119	128	136	145	153
55	165	99	107	116	124	132	140	149
60	160	96	104	112	120	128	136	144
65	155	93	101	109	116	124	132	140
70	150	90	97	105	113	120	128	135
75	145	87	94	102	109	116	123	131
80	140	84	91	98	105	112	119	126
85	135	81	88	95	101	108	115	122

12 Week Aerobic Program

Workout	# 1 %Hrm/time	# 2 %Hrm/time	# 3 % Hr/time
Week 1	60/15	60/15	60/15
Week 2	60/20	60/15	60/20
Week 3	60/20	60/15	60/15
Week 4	60/20	60/20	60/20
Week 5	65/20	65/20	65/20
Week 6	65/20	60/20	60/20
Week 7	65/20	65/20	70/20
Week 8	70/20	65/20	70/20
Week 9	70/20	65/20	65/20
Week 10	70/20	70/20	70/20
Week 11	75/20	75/20	70/20
Week 12	75/20	75/20	75/20

TEN

Testing For Maximum Strength

In many classical exercise texts, the term "maximum strength" is often referred to as the highest force or tension generated by a muscle or muscle group during a voluntary maximum contraction. Developing testing procedures to determine an individual's maximum strength hasn't always been a high priority in sports and fitness. It wasn't until fairly recently that measuring maximum strength levels took on any significance at all.

Prior to the late 1960s, only those individuals involved in competitive weightlifting, bodybuilding and a small number of isolated sports needed to know their exact strength levels on a periodic basis. For the rest of the general fitness and athletic public, there was little reason to have an accurate process for measuring strength. This unfortunate situation existed because of the belief that using weight training to increase strength levels caused "muscle boundness". Even as late as the 1980s, many top fitness experts in the United States completely ignored strength training as part of a complete fitness program.

In our new age of enlightenment we know that using progressive resistance weight training to increase strength levels provides an individual with an array of benefits including; decreasing the risk of athletic injuries, increasing the recovery rate in various sports related injuries, increasing athletic speed, increasing athletic power, motor agility and muscular endurance. With all these benefits, it is imperative that we have an accurate system for testing a persons maximum strength levels.

Currently there are four general ways to measure muscular strength. They are: tensiometry, dynamometry, computer determined force/work output and the one repetition maximum (1-RM). Tensiometry involves using an instrument called a tensiometer. This instrument (which was originally designed to test cable strengths for various airplane sections) measures muscular force during the static contractions of a muscle. Dynamometry also employs the use of an instrument called a dynamometer. There are a couple of kinds of these devices but all operate by using static compression to measure the force of the working muscle.

As the name implies, computer determined force/work output is measured with the help of a computer which can accurately determine the muscular force generated by the muscle during a variety of movements as well as during several phases of an individual exercise.

Finally, the 1-RM is the maximal weight load a person is capable of lifting for one repetition of an exercise. Of all four ways of testing, the 1-RM is the most realistic and efficient strength test for most people to use in a typical gym setting. The reason it's so realistic is that you do not need any special instruments, devices or computers to perform a 1-RM strength test; any type of typical gym equipment will do. Also, a 1-RM may be performed on any exercise whether it's a leg press, bench press or shoulder press.

Before you run off to the gym to bang out 1-RMs, there are some important principles on how to take a proper, accurate and above all safe 1-RM. To begin, remember that taking a 1-RM is not meant to be an all out powerlifting event where the end justifies the means. Never sacrifice lifting form for higher weight loads. Perfect lifting form must be used on each of the testing exercises, without exception. Cheating by throwing the weight load up or wiggling and juggling until you complete the 1-RM may help your ego, but it will also increase your potential for injury as well as give you a false reading of your strength levels. That can spell disaster, especially if you're using an advance training program like "phase training". Therefore make sure you spend some time perfecting your lifting technique before you perform your 1-RM. Also make sure that your training partner doesn't help you perform the testing repetition by using a forced rep. Any assistance in performing the 1-RM nullifies the result.

Remember that regardless of what piece of equipment you're testing on, always have a spotter. Never test alone! This is especially true if you're using free weights. Many times you'll be using testing loads which may be higher than you would normally use, so you'll want to make sure there's somebody around. Make sure, too, that your 1-RM testing follows the same workout pattern as your normal workout routine. In other words, if you train your chest, shoulders and triceps together in one work-out, test them the same day and in the same order. Do not test your chest exercises one day and your shoulders the next if you usually work them together.

In order to perform a correct 1-RM test, it's imperative that you begin the testing workout, with a complete warm-up period. This includes both a general warm-up, followed by a specific warm-up. The general warm-up may be any aerobic activity you prefer. A general warm-up should be between fifteen to twenty-five minutes at a moderate intensity level, and again, any moderate activity will do; calisthenics, running, skipping rope, bike riding, or playing basketball.

The specific warm-up is performed in a circuit manner on all your testing exercises for one or two sets. Use about thirty to thirty-five percent of your present maximal weight load capacity for twenty or more repetitions. These light loads will allow your neuromuscular system to begin anticipating the exact exercise movement that you'll be performing your 1-RM.
After you're warmed-up, the weight load pattern for test-

ing each exercise should follow the classical pyramid method. This means that as you progress from one set to another, you add weight as you decrease the repetitions. On the first set, always start with a submaximal weight load which allows you to easily perform twelve to fifteen repetitions. On the second set, you may add anywhere from five to twenty percent increases in weight load (depending on your lifting experience) and perform a set of ten to twelve reps.

Repeat this pattern of increasing weight loads and decreasing reps for several sets until you reach a set in which you're only able to complete one perfect rep. That set would be recorded as your 1-RM. For accurate testing, it's important to note that the rest intervals (RI) between testing sets should increase as your weight loads increase. On the first couple of sets, your RI may be around two minutes, but as you approach your maximum lifts the RI may be up five to seven minutes. The longer RIs are necessary to allow the body complete muscular and neuromuscular recovery between sets.

Finally, because of the extended warm-ups, sets and RIs involved in testing, the 1-RM workout(s) will take longer than your normal workout, so plan ahead. Remember, too, that testing for maximum strength is a tool which is used to help plan out your future workouts. Do not abuse this tool. Performing 1-RM testing should be used sparingly, depending upon your experience, motivation and type of training program. In general, testing for maximum strength should be performed two to three a year for beginners, four times a year for intermediates, and up to five times a year for advanced (non-competitive) individuals.

Choose always the way that seems best, however rough it may be. Custom will soon render it easy and agreeable

ELEVEN

Designing Your Workout "Body-Part Grouping"

In setting up your workouts you must be aware that it takes up to 48 to 72 hours for a muscle to recover from training stress, after it has been sufficiently worked. It should be understood that you cannot work a muscle or its supporting muscles two days in a row. Supporting muscle is one that is used in some form of support for the main or core muscle being worked.

An example is the interaction between the chest, shoulders and triceps. The chest is the core muscle group, while the shoulders and triceps are supportive muscle groups. Knowing this, you cannot work the chest on Monday, and then work shoulders and triceps on Tuesday since any time you do chest work, like bench pressing, you are also using your shoulders and triceps .

Hitting shoulders the day after benching does not supply adequate recovery time for the shoulders. If you follow this kind of routine, your shoulders become overly fatigued and won't be trained efficiently. This is why many people complain that they are not strong in the shoulders when they work them the day of benching. This concept applies for back and biceps work as well. The back cannot be exercised on one day and biceps the following day because they work together.

Another point in setting up the structure of your workouts is that a muscle needs to be worked two times per week in order to adapt it to that week's training load before an increase in weight load is made. It has been accepted by experts that a muscle begins to weaken approximately 6 days after a workout. Routines that hit each body part once a week cannot properly stress the body's system for adaptation . Remember, we want to work a muscle and then let it rest so it can adapt and regenerate. Contrary to popular belief, this does not mean you have to be strong each day.

Now that you understand the criteria of body part grouping, it is time to pick the number of days a week you plan to workout. You want to hit each body part at least twice a week with the proper grouping. It is recommended that your selection of days be dependent on how many times per week you want to, or have time to, workout.

Be realistic in your selection of days. If your time schedule dictates 4 days a week, then go with that. Save yourself frustration by not making conflicting goals with your training schedule. Conflicting training goals begin by trying to fit more workouts in per week than you have time for. This will cause you to miss too many workouts.

OUTLINE:

1) Do not work a body part or its supporting muscle 2 days in a row. Allow the muscle the proper time to rest and regenerate.

2) Do not create a program in which you work each body part once a week .Train each bodypart at least 2x per week or 3x in a 2 week cycle.

3) Stay away from mood training. Stick to your plan.

4) Do not make conflicting goals with your workout schedule. Be realistic about the time you have each week to train.

TWELVE

Circuit Training

Time, when you think about it, time is a precious, non-renewable commodity which, unfortunately, all of us take for granted. The commodity of time, like many other commodities, comes in units of measurements; years, months, weeks, days, hours, minutes, seconds and so on. These units give us a reference point of where it is we stand in our relative existence.

In every 24 hour period, regardless of what time zone you're in you're given 86,400 seconds of your commodity of time to invest into the activities of that day. If you've made a decision to invest some of those seconds into a training program for strength, general fitness, aerobic conditioning or body development, then you should learn how to invest your precious investment seconds wisely. Remember, in the gym time may be either a trusted ally working with you to help you reach your goals, or it can be your enemy keeping you bogged down in a quagmire.

If you're pressed for workout time, but want to reap the benefits of a training program for both strength, fitness and aerobic improvement, you may want to consider a method of training called "circuit training". Circuit training which is also called *circuit resistance training* (CRT) is not a new or revolutionary idea by any means. It has been around, and used quite successfully for a number of years by fitness and medical experts.

Many equipment companies such as Nautilus, Cybex and Universal design exercise equipment specifically to be used in a circuit program. Even though the CRT methods and equipment have been in existence for some time, their potential and use as a mainstay method of training has not been fully exploited. Why this situation is allowed to exist is something which is hard to understand.

Besides its time saving benefits, a CRT program has been shown to increase aerobic capabilities and strength levels in individuals who use a CRT program consistently. A properly designed CRT program is an excellent off season transitional training method for athletes, and when modified, it can be a superb warm-up routine prior to a more traditional training program. Also, a CRT program which is supervised medically has been shown to be effective in the improvement of various medical conditions, specifically coronary, cardiac and spinal cord injured conditions.

The idea behind circuit training is relatively simple, it combines aerobic conditioning and strength conditioning in one training period. The aerobic conditioning is established by keeping the heart rate raised during the entire workout, and the strength conditioning is established by using progressive resistance. This dual act is accomplished by training your entire body in one workout, 2 to 3 times per week. The accompanying exercises on an circuit program are performed one after another with various rest intervals (RI) used between exercises.

As with any methodology of exercise and fitness training, there are many variations of CRT training. A typical circuit program may be any where from 20 to 50 minutes in total workout length, encompassing 7 to 15 exercises. In a classical CRT program, you move from one exercise to another without stopping. At the end of one complete circuit you would repeat another circuit, and depending on your ability level and condition, you may perform 2 to 4 complete circuits. A variation on the classical non-stop method is to have a RI of approximately 15 to 30 seconds between each exercise (more about this method later).

In a CRT program, there can be variations for the

loading pattern for weight loads and reps. The first school of thought uses time as a determining factor. Here a trainee would set the weight load for each exercise at approximately 40% to 55% of their one repetition maximum (a 1-RM is the maximum weight load a trainee could lift for one repetition either actual or calculated).

The weight load for each exercise would then be performed for a period of time, let's say 15 seconds in a rhythmic lifting pattern. As the trainee improves in performance, the time for lifting the weight loads would increase per exercise, perhaps eventually up to 30 seconds. If you're using a method which allows for rest in between exercises, then the basic ratio between exercise performance and rest would be 1:1. A 15 second exercise performance would be followed by a 15 second rest period before the next exercise would begin, this pattern would repeat itself throughout the workout. Beginners may want to use a 1:2 ratio were the RI would be double of that of the performance interval, until a level of adaptability is achieved.

A second loading pattern for weight loads and reps follow the more traditional pattern of increasing weight loads as the reps decrease progressively from one circuit to another. This traditional pattern would start the first circuit at a weight load which allows the trainee to perform an exercise for 12 to 15 reps per exercise. The weight loads in the second circuit would then be increased as the reps decrease. Therefore the second set would then use an increased weight load which would allow a trainee to perform an exercise for 10 reps, and depending upon the program design the third set to increase weight load to allow for only 8 reps per exercise.

If you're using the traditional progressive resistance pattern for circuit training, the pattern for the weight loads and reps would be based on the goals and level of ability of the individual training on the program.

Regardless of which weight load pattern you use, the exercise pattern for a circuit program should be based on alternating muscle groups, with the size of the muscle group being the determining factor. In other words, you would begin you're circuit with the largest muscle group, your leg exercises.

The leg exercises would alternate with work performed by your back, chest, shoulders, arms and abdominals respectively. This type of exercise pattern follows a more natural and logical flow to a workout than a haphazard exercise patterns.

Many gyms which have a circuit area, the CRT machines are not always set-up in an easy to follow pattern. Many of the machines are scattered, helter skelter which tends to leave the trainee who may not be fully aware of how to use them quite confused. Some exercise patterns which may start with a leg exercise then move directly to arms, then to back, to shoulders then to abs. The problem with this type of random pattern is that if you perform an arm exercise, let's say tricep extensions, and then you move to a chest exercise i.e. bench press, the efficiency of the bench press is compromised.

This compromise occurs because your triceps our a supportive muscle group for the chest, therefore if they are fatigued, they cannot perform effectively as they should in supporting your chest exercise. This holds true for shoulders which also support the chest, the biceps which support the back, and so on. Leaving the abs and low back for last allows for complete recovery of the other major muscle groups before you hit them again on another circuit.

A well designed CRT program would begin with a 10 - 15 minute aerobic warm-up performed on a treadmill, stationary bike or some make of step climber.

The following are two CRT workouts, one is based on 4 major primary exercises, and the second is expanded to include not only the primary exercises, but also secondary exercises.

Workout 1

Aerobic warm-up.

Exercise:
1. Leg Press
2. Pulldown
3. Bench Press
4. Ab Crunch

Pattern - Leg Press - Pulldown - Bench Press - Ab Crunch .

Workout 2

Aerobic warm-up

Exercises:
1. Leg Press
2. Leg Extension
3. Leg Curl
4. Pulldown
5. Bench Press
6. Military Press
7. Tricep Extension
8. Biceps Curl
9. Ab Crunch

Pattern : Leg Press - Curl Grip Pulldown - Leg Curl - Bench Press -Leg Extension - Shoulder Press - Bicep Curls - Tricep Pulldowns -Ab Crunch.

Using workout 1 and 2 as a working base model incorporating the outlines previously mentioned in regard to the weight load patterns, you can begin to create various other models depending upon your specific needs and goals. Make a note that CRT can be a very dynamic method of training which may take some getting use to. If you're new to this form of training, it would be a good idea to start at a slow pace, with limited exercises and expand from there. Also if you feel the need to stop at any point during a CRT program to "catch your breath", then by all means do. As with all training programs, use your common sense and allow your body to gradually adapt to new training program and new levels of intensities.

NOTE: See Chapter Twenty-Five for Exercise Descriptions

Designing Your Circuit Training Program Notes

_____
_____
_____
_____
_____
_____
_____
_____
_____
_____
_____
_____
_____
_____
_____
_____
_____

THIRTEEN

Peripheral Heart Training

If reaping the myriad benefits of an exercise and fitness program is important to you, there is a terrific and efficient training method called "Peripheral Heart Training" (PHT). Using and understanding the following principles of a PHT program will insure that your precious training hours aren't wasted off-handed.

Although Peripheral Heart Training may sound like an exotic methodology, it isn't as complex as it sounds. Actually, Peripheral Heart Training is a simple idea which finds its foundation in CRT which was discussed in the previous chapter.

There are several similarities and benefits between these two fitness training methods. For example, both PHT and CRT involve combining cardio-vascular conditioning and strength conditioning in one training session. Both depend on working the entire body in one workout. Both may be performed with free weights or machines. Lastly, both can be very dynamic and time saving.

Unlike classical CRT though, the object behind a PHT program is to train selective muscle groups together using three or four exercises in one "mini-circuit". Several of these mini-circuits are then put together to form one complete total body workout. As you perform these PHT mini-circuits, blood is sent racing rapidly from one part of the body to another, working the cardiovascular system. At the same time, you push various weight loads using core exercises, thereby taxing your strength system.

On a PHT program, a mini-circuit would start with a lower body exercise. From there, you would go directly to a mid-body exercise and end with an upper body exercise. Once the mini-circuit was complete, you would begin the same circuit over again. When the number of predetermined sets on your program are completed, you would begin your next mini-circuit of three alternating exercises and so on. These smaller circuits allow you to focus more intensely on the primary core exercises before you move on to the secondary muscle groups.

As you perform a PHT circuit, the weight load pattern, sets and repetitions all depend on your PHT program design. Many PHT programs employ the traditional weight loading pattern of increased weight loads with decreasing repetitions as you progress from one set to another, but this is not written in stone. As stated before, cardiovascular and strength conditioning would be the foundational combined goals, but there are many other specific training effects which could be designed into a PHT program. These specific training effects could include a combination of; muscle-endurance, power, physique definition, muscle-hypertrophy and muscle fiber-type combination training as well.

To get started on a good solid and basic PHT program, you would want to design the program for three training sessions in a seven day period. Each workout consists of your core exercises for each body part. These exercises would include:

Legs - leg press, leg extension, leg curl, calf raises.
Back - pulldown, low back.
Chest - bench press.
Shoulders - military press.
Triceps - tricep extension.
Biceps - bicep curls.
Abdominals - ab crunch, ab crunch twist.

Training Days: Monday-Wednesday-Friday

PHT circuit 1.

Leg Press	=	set#1x15 - #2x12 - #3x10 - #4x8
Ab Crunch	=	set#1x15 - #2x15 - #3x15 - #4x15
Lat Pulldown	=	set#1x15 - #2x10 - #3x10 - #4x8

Note: If you're using moderate or maximal weight loads, you may need to take a few extra seconds to rest in between rounds of each mini-circuit. This pattern of extended rest intervals would apply to each mini-circuit on your PHT program.

PHT circuit 2.

Leg Extension	=	set#1x12 - #2x10 - #3x10 - #4x8
Ab Twist	=	set#1x15 - #2x15 - #3x15 - #4x15
Bench Press	=	set#1x15 - #2x12- #3x10 - #4x8

PHT circuit 3.

Leg Curl	=	set#1x12 - #2x10 - #3x10 - #4x8
Low Ab Crunch	=	set#1x10 - #2x10 - #3x10 - #4x10
Military Press	=	set#1x15 - #2x10 - #3x10 - #4x8

After you have completed your last Shoulder Press set in mini-circuit #3, move directly to your next mini-circuit.

PHT circuit 4.
Calf Raise	=	set#1x15 - #2x10 - #3x10 - #4x8
Tricep Pushdown	=	set#1x15 - #2x12 - #3x10 - #4x8
Bicep Curl	=	set#1x15 - #2x12 - #3x10 - #4x8

If you have never used any type of circuit training before, especially a PHT circuit program, give yourself some time and let your body adapt to this dynamic training method gradually.

FOURTEEN

The Sixty Minute Working Person's Workout

Congratulations. You finally made it to the big time. You're a high power executive in a heavy hitting company, living in the city that never sleeps. Your day-to-day life is filled with meetings, business dinners, handling dozens of problems and making decision after decision. This whole process begins about 7:00am and usually ends about 8:00pm. That is unless you have a last minute deadline, or the clients from Japan want to go out for drinks. Even with the fast pace and pressure, you enjoy your work and wouldn't trade it for anything.

There is one problem though. Lately you've noticed that your energy levels just aren't what they use to be. You feel tried, sluggish and heavy. And your stomach. Man! What use to be flat is now beginning to resemble some kind of weird statue of Buddha. The bottom line is, you just don't like the way you look or feel anymore. You know the answer to correcting these challenges is an exercise conditioning program. Unfortunately, you just do not have the time. Does the scenario sound familiar?

If you're a professional business executive, you owe it to yourself, your future, your family and your career to increase your level of physical fitness. The excuse of not having enough time to train may be legitimate, but it doesn't change anything. The simple fact is that one way or another, you have to make the time to exercise. Remember, you made the time to do all the things that got you where you are today. You can find the time to exercise. And the best place to start is at lunch time.

Lunch time training has many benefits. First, the sixty minutes usually scheduled for lunch is already logged in most people's daily plan. Replacing those sixty minutes of eating and drinking with working out three times a week is not a drastic lifestyle change. Also, with sixty minutes planned for training, no time can be wasted flapping your jaw. You have to get in and get out. This means very effective and efficient workouts. Lunch time workouts also gives you a positive break in your day, allowing you get away from it all for a short time. When you get back to the office you'll feel good, your energy levels will be soaring, and your positive mental attitude will be sky-high.

In designing a sixty minute workout, three different training aspects need consideration for a complete conditioning program. These three aspects are aerobic training, strength conditioning and flexibility training. Also, a warm-up and cool down period will also be included as sub-components of your program. As you progress through your program, your ability to increase intensities will vary with each aspect.

Aerobic training takes the longest amount of time to safely increase training intensities, strength takes a shorter amount of time, and finally flexibility takes the shortest. The workout pattern for this sixty minute workout will be three workouts per week. Training three days will produce excellent training results while providing you the plenty of rest time in-between workouts. Your off training days could be spent participating in some sport to provided added training and health benefits.

The pattern for a three day workout week will follow a Monday, Wednesday and Friday rotation. Take note that you'll be performing two different workouts on this program. Workout A will consist of training the legs, and and biceps, and workout B will consist of training the chest, shoulders and triceps. Since two different workouts will be used in this program, we'll need to rotate workouts every week so that in every two week period each body part will be trained 3 times. An example of this rotating pattern would be: Week one workouts / A, B, A. Week two workouts / B, A, B.

Since you are limited in your training time, we'll choose the most effective exercises for each body part. Remember that you do not have to do dozens of exercise to produce results. For this program, you'll be using the most effective compound exercises for each body part. Compound exercises are exercises which use not only the main muscle of a body part, put also work the supportive group of muscle. The reason for choosing compound exercises is that these exercises create the greatest demands on the body for the fastest results. The following exercises will be used as the foundation of your sixty minute workout.

Workout A

1. Legs / leg press and leg curl
2. Back / lat pulldown
3. Biceps / dumbbell curls

Workout B

1.Chest / bench press
2.Shoulders / military press
3.Triceps / extensions

Let's start to put all the components together along with some reference times. You may need to make some adjustments to fit your particular situation. Even though many corporations nowadays have either an in-house training facility, or are located near a gym, it may take some added time to get to the gym.

Minutes 0-20 : The first period of your program will consist of the aerobic portion of the training. This period will also act as a warm-up. For your aerobic conditioning period, choose any aerobic activity you enjoy doing. Treadmill, stationary bike, step climber all are excellent pieces of equipment. You may want to choose a different piece of aerobic equipment for workout A & B. Start by performing your aerobics period with low intensity level. Increases in intensity levels should only be made in every two week cycle.

Minutes 20-25 : At the completion of the aerobic period, an easy flexibility conditioning period will be performed. Remember, flexibility conditioning or stretching, is always performed after the warm-up never before. Start your flexibility period from the head and work your way down. This way you do not have to keep getting up and down off the floor. Make sure you add the flexibility period in every workout. Gains in flexibility can be made from workout to workout.

Minutes 25-50: At the completion of you five minutes flexibility period, you can start your strength conditioning period. By this time in your workout, you should be properly warmed-up so that adding a specific warm-up period will not be needed. Start all your exercises with a set of twelve to fifteen repetitions using moderate weight load, about fifty-five percent of you maximum weight loads. Form there you can increase loads as you lower the reps. As you near the last exercises on your program, begin to shake your arms out, roll your shoulders and so on. These small movements will act as a cool down period which will help your muscles eliminate waste by products from the workout and help to begin the recovery process.

Minutes 50-60: Shower and change.

FIFTEEN

Cycling Phase Training

What is *cycling*? Cycling training (also known as phase training or periodization) simply means varying and changing the different aspects of your training program on a constant and regular basis. On a cycled weight training program, aspects like, weight loads, sets, reps, rest intervals, duration and frequency of workouts are periodically changed in order to keep any one system of the body from being overworked for too long.

Using cycles of training is not a new concept , it has been used successfully in athletic training for sports for decades. Many people stumble across this pattern of training accidentally. This usually occurs after they've hit a training plateau and feel the need for a change. The inner feeling of needing a change in training is a normal event, because it follows the natural cycles of the body. There are a few basic factors to consider in cycling body-building training.

The first factor to consider is the level of will power and training experience of the individual. As stated previously, no two people are the same. They differ in their genetic make-up, muscle fiber type combination, motivational powers, recovery powers, the ability to accept pain, the ability to focus and so on. All these factors dictate how long each individual can safely stay on one cycle of training before moving to another cycle.

Some individuals because of sheer will power and experience can sustain a longer amount of time on a very stressfull high intensity cycle that would wear down someone else. This individual "right stuff" of a person's character must be understood before a cycling program begins.

The next factor in cycling training program is the intensity ranges for each of the individual cycles. Intensity ranges are not randomly chosen, there are some basic guidelines to be followed. Generally, there are three major cycles that a person should experience. Light intensity cycles, moderate intensity cycles and high intensity cycles. These cycles can be strung together in an endless variation of combinations as long as the before mentioned "right stuff" is taken into account.

Light intensity cycles may be used anytime a person feels that they are worn out from heavy training. These cycles may also be used after a competition to allow the body to cool down from being in competitive shape, or they may be used to get into pre-training shape after a long lay off or injury, and they may even be used if a person just wants to stay active while planning their future training goals.

In light cycle training, weight loads between 45 to 70 percent of your maximal lifting ability are used. The repetition range may be anywhere from 10 to 15 reps depending upon the weight load, and the rest interval between sets should be around 1 to 2 minutes. The duration of a light cycle may be anywhere from 4 to 8 weeks.

Next , moderate cycles of training intensities allows a person to achieve spurts in muscles size. Moderate cycles use weight loads between 70 to 80 percent of a persons maximal lifting ability. The repetition range in a moderate cycle may be from 8 to 10 reps for 4 to 5 sets. Here, rest intervals need to be a bit longer than in a light cycle, perhaps up to 3 minutes between sets. The duration of moderate cycles of training may be anywhere from 8 to 12 weeks before a switch over to a different cycle is needed.

Finally, high intensity training cycles are used to allow an individual to develop a greater degree of density to their muscles. High intensity cycles are usually the shortest cycles lasting only four to six weeks before a change is made. The heaviest weight loads of any cycle will be used here. Loads as high has 85 to 95 percent of maximal lifting ability may be used. On the other end, the repetition ranges will be the lowest, anywhere from four to six reps depending upon the weight load with rest intervals between sets approximately four or five minutes.

If you're considering cycling your training, use the outlines mentioned here as a starting point but remember, one cycling program will work for everyone. Each of our "right stuff" is different, so some experimentation is needed to find out what will work best for you. Also, keep exact records of all the weight loads, sets and reps on your program in order to have some data to draw from, as you arrange your future cycles. And finally, change is good, but not every week or workout to workout. Give your body time to adapt and improve on one cycle of training before you change to another.

Lesson Notes: Plan out a 12 week cycling training program using light, moderate and high intensity cycles.

_____
_____
_____
_____
_____
_____
_____
_____
_____
_____
_____
_____
_____
_____

REVIEW QUESTIONS

A. Explain the importance of a proper warm up before a workout.

_____
_____
_____
_____
_____
_____
_____

B. List eight stretches a person should NOT do.

1._____   5._____
2._____   6._____
3._____   7._____
4._____   8._____

C. Explain the role aerobic training plays in an overall fitness program.

_____
_____
_____
_____
_____
_____
_____
_____
_____
_____
_____
_____

D. Calculate your Predicted Maximum Heart Rate.
HRM_____

E. List four ways to test a persons strength level.

1._____

2._____

3._____

4._____

F. Explain how to take a 1Rm strength test.

_____

_____

_____

_____

_____

_____

_____

_____

_____

G. Explain the difference between CRT and PHT fitness training.

_____

_____

_____

_____

_____

_____

_____

_____

H. What is Cycling Training?

_____

_____

_____

_____

_____

_____

SIXTEEN

Cycling
Phase One
ACTIVATION

In phase training activation is always the first phase on any plan regardless of the final outcome. This is a phase used to prepare your body for the demands of the harder training. Your supporting structures such as your ligaments, tendons, muscles, and nervous system are the primary targets of this phase. Activation has an added benefit because it increases your chance for injury-free training, and helps recovery from other training systems which may have caused overtraining.

In essence "Activation" means to alert, involve and fire-up the body. This type of training is multilateral. Affecting the muscular system to enhance strength, the cardio-respiratory system (CR) systems (heart and respiratory systems that work together to supply oxygen to the body and remove carbon dioxide) to strengthen your heart and improve circulation, and the nervous system to facilitate the ability of your muscles to be enlisted quickly and completely.

The cardio-respiratory endurance work in this phase can be performed separately or as a warm up for your strength work. Continuous, moderately intense exercise for 10-20 minutes on a bike, treadmill or steppers is all that is needed during this phase. Moreover, it can be a very effective and efficient means of warming up. The activation phase is so important that no person should skip this phase regardless of experience and ability.

During activation, the weight loads used are not too demanding on the body. The weight loads you lift during this phase should be comfortable. Too much discomfort due to trying to lift very heavy weights before your body's systems are prepared (activated) is one of the primary causes of overtraining and injuries. You will be doing up to 15 reps during a set during the activation phase, and if you are not accustomed to this many repetitions you may find this challenging but not demanding.

Lighter weights used during this phase allows your body to accustom itself to being challenged with training stress. The lighter weights are also particularly applicable to developing connective tissues such as ligament and tendon. Of course, while using lighter weights you should also be concentrating very intensely on correct lifting technique, using the proper muscles, and moving through complete range of motion. Developing perfect lifting technique is an extremely important aspect of the Activation phase and one that must not be neglected. Concentrating on techniques will work the muscles through a complete and full range of motion, totally adapting the muscles, tendons and ligaments for the work to come.

If you are accustomed to lifting heavy weights you are likely to feel like you are not working hard enough during this phase. Among people who have used cycling training programs, this phase is often called "guilt training", because you don't feel like you're "gutting-it-out." However, rest assured that you are laying a vital foundation for your future progress, and be patient. Remember, the scope of the training at this point is to reactivate and readjust all your internal systems.

This reactivating is especially true for the neuromuscular system (nerve and muscle coordinating system). As a result of good adaptation, the muscle fiber firing rate also increases. This means that when more fibers are activated, a person sees good results.

Program Recommendations

1. Calculate your workloads. Perform a 1RM test record your results

2. Calculate your percentages of the 1RM. Use this simple equation to find your weight loads: your 1RM x Percentage / 100 = the weight load. Example : Bench Press RM = 200 lbs. X 45/100 = 90 lbs. Or 200 x .45 = 90 lbs. Use this procedure for all your exercises. Take your time in your calculations, make sure to use the correct percentages for the exercises.

As you examine the percentage formulas in Table 1. You'll see they are designed for beginners, intermediates and advanced athletes. If you're just starting out or have less then one year of strength training, use beginner formulas. If you have over one year strength training experience, use that experience to select the intermediate

ACTIVATION Beginner

	Set 1	Set 2	Set 3
Week # 1	45% x 15	50 % x 12	50 % x 12
Week # 2	45 % x 15	50 % x 15	50 % x 15
Week # 3	45 % x 15	50 % x 15	60 % x 10
Week # 4	45 % x 15	50 % x 12	60 % x 8

ACTIVATION Intermediate / Advanced

	Set 1	Set 2	Set 3	Set4
Week # 1	45% x 15	50 % x 12	50 % x 12	60 % x 10
Week # 2	45 % x 15	50 % x 15	50 % x 15	60 % x 10
Week # 3	45 % x 15	50 % x 15	60 % x 10	65 % x 10
Week # 4	45 % x 15	50 % x 12	60 % x 8	60 % x 10

SEVENTEEN

Cycling
Phase Two
STRENGTH

The next phase in a cycling program is strength. As a rule this phase should follow activation. The main training goals of this phase are:

1. To increase muscular strength.
2. To increase the tone of muscles.
3. To increase recruitment of fast twitch muscle fibers.

The initial physiological response that occurs during the strength phase is neurological. Using near maximal weight loads (70-90% of your 1RMXs) facilitates the nervous system to recruit more muscle fibers. For example when you lift near maximal weight loads with few reps (1-6) the nervous system "fires" recruiting an increased number of additional muscle fibers to allow you to complete your set. As you train through this phase more and more previously "asleep" muscle fibers will be recruited. These newly recruited muscle fibers will then be called up in later phases of training.

True gains in strength and muscle density are the direct result of neuromuscular adaptation and a rise in the protein content of the muscle. Increasing the protein content of the muscle increases a persons ability to lift higher weight loads, thereby becoming stronger.

Using weight loads from 70-90% creates an excellent partnership between the nervous system and muscular system. These loads stimulate a call to arms between these two systems by improving their "signals" which in turn "fires up" more muscle fibers.

Also, heavy loads are necessary to develop higher levels of tension within the muscle. This increase tension is an important aspect in developing maximum strength and ultimately muscle density. Therefore, this increased density leads to more muscle tone.

The strength phase is very demanding and will have you lifting much heavier weight loads than you did during the activation phase. It is very important that you do not skip the activation phase because it should have prepared your body for the greater workloads that you will encounter during the strength phase. Also, when you enter this second phase you should have perfected your lifting techniques allowing for optimal progress and injury free training.

As with with all cycling programs this phase incorporates the step-load pattern. This means that you perform two progression-block weeks followed by a down loading week. Remember that at the end of week four of activation a new 1RMX was determined. These new RMXs are used to calculate the workload percentages for the strength phase.

Strength Workout
Beginner

Week	Set 1	Set 2	Set 3
1	60 % x 12	70 % x 8	80 % x 6
2	60 % x 12	70 % x 8	85 % x 4-5
3	60 % x 12	75 % x 6	75 % x 6
4	60 % x 10	75 % x 8	85 % x4
5	65 % x 10	85 % x 5	90 % x 3
6	65 % x 10	75 % x 8	80 % x 4

Test on the first workout of week five. It is considered a workout in itself. Continue on week five as soon as you calculate your new weight loads.

Strength Workout
Intermediate

Week	Set 1	Set 2	Set 3	Set 4
1	55% x 12	70% x 8	75% x 6	75% x 6
2	55% x 12	70% x 8	80% x 4	85% x 3
3	55% x 12	70% x 8	75% x 6	75% x 6
4	60% x 10	75% x 8	85% x 3	90% x 2-
5	50% x 10	80% x 4	85% x 3	90% x 2
6	60% x 10	75% x 6	80% x 4	80% x 4

Test on the first workout of week five. It is considered a workout in itself. Continue on week five as soon as you calculate your new weight loads.

Strength Workout
Advanced

Week	Set 1	Set 2	Set 3	Set 4	Set 5
1	55% x 10	70% x 8	75% x 8	80% x 6	80% x 6
2	55% x 10	75% x 8	80% x 6	80% x 6	85% x 4
3	55% x 10	70% x 8	75% x 6	75% x 6	80% x 4
4	55% x 10	75% x8	85% x 4	85% x 4	90% x 3
5	55% x 10	75% x 8	85% x 4	90% x 2	90% x 3
6	55% x 10	75% x 6	75% x 6	80% x 4	80% x 4

Test on the first workout of week five. It is considered a workout in itself. Continue on week five as soon as you calculate your new weight loads.

When you end the strength development phase you have the option to perform another strength phase, repeat an activation phase or begin a new phase - development.

EIGHTEEN

Cycling Phase Three Muscle Hypertrophy

The next phase of a cycling program is muscle hypertrophy. As a rule this phase should follow a strength development phase. The main training goals of this phase are:

1. To increase the size of muscle fibers.
2. Stimulate increases in muscular capillaries.
3. Increase bone mass.
4. Possibly increase the number of muscle fibers (hyperplasia).

Remember, in this phase, we are trying to develop highly functional lean body weight and not highly un-usable body fat.

The duration of the muscle hypertrophy phase is between six and twelve weeks. During these phases weight loads and repetitions are geared toward develop-ing "hypertrophy" or muscle growth . The weight loads in this phase vary from 65% to 85% of your 1RM using 6-10 repetitions, respectively.

In order to understand muscle hypertrophy, let us examine the anatomy and physiology of muscular devel-opment. Skeletal muscle is an extremely dynamic tissue with an impressive capacity to adapt both anatomically and physiologically. Heavy resistance training results in an increase in cross-sectional area of contractile protein. Interstitial connective tissue also increases in proportion to the increase in fiber area.

While some researches have suggested that weight training may also result in an increase in fiber number in adult muscle, this general belief is that fiber number is established at birth and no net increase will occur during your mass development phase. However, skeletal muscle also possesses a population of reserve or satellite cells, which, when activated can trigger a sequence of events that result in the replacement of damaged fibers with new fibers.

During the muscle hypertrophy phase "stressed" fibers will be replaced by satellite fibers. Simply stated, muscle growth is a chain of chemical reactions that occur as a result of its reaction to resistance training. It is the muscles reactions to stress. A muscle grows to protect itself from this stress. The muscle will mobilize its resources so that it can increase its ability to withstand the physical challenges of training. Following the stress of training your muscle requires rest. You must rest adequately (48-72 hrs) for your muscles to grow and before you can "shock" them again.

As with the first and second phase of cycling training, this phase incorporates the step-load pattern. This means that you perform two progression weeks followed by a down loading week. Remember that at the end of week 4 of the strength phase a new RMX was determined. These new RMX's are used to calculate the workload percentages for the muscle hypertrophy phase.

Muscle Hypertrophy Workout Beginner

Week	Set 1	Set 2	Set 3	Set 4
1	55% X 10	65% X 8	70% X 6	70% X 6
2	55% X 10	65% X 8	75% X 6	75% X 6
3	55% X 10	65% X 8	70% X 6	70% X 6
4	55% X 10	65% X 10	70% X 8	75% X 6
5	55% X 10	70% X 8	75% X 6	75% X 6
6	55% X 10	65% X 10	70% X 6	75% X 6

Test on the first workout at the beginning of week 7, then continue using the sane workouts that you did in week 6 to finish week 7.

Muscle Hypertrophy Workout Intermediate

Week	Set 1	Set 2	Set 3	Set 4
1	55% X 10	65% X 8	70% X 6	70% X 6
2	55% X 10	65% X 8	70% X 8	75% X 6
3	55% X 10	65% X 10	65% X 8	70% X 6
4	55% X 10	65% X 8	70% X 8	70% X 8
5	55% X 10	70% X 8	75% X 6	75% X 6
6	55% X 10	65% X 8	70% X 8	70% X 6

Muscle Hypertrophy Workout Advanced

Week	Set 1	Set 2	Set 3	Set 4	Set 5
1	55% X 10	65% X 8	65% X 8	70% X 6	70% X 6
2	55% X 10	65% X 8	65% X 10	70% X 8	75% X 6
3	55% X 10	65% X 8	65% X 8	70% X 6	70% X 6
4	55% X 10	70% X 8	70% X 8	75% X 6	75% X 6
5	55% X 10	70% X 8	70% X 8	75% X 6	80% X 6
6	55% X 10	65% X 8	70% X 8	75% X 6	75% X 6

Test on the first workout at the beginning of week 7, then continue using the same workouts that you did in week 6 to finish week 7.

When you complete the mass development phase you have the option to perform another mass phase if your goal is to increase size or to begin a new phase. "Definition", look for this phase in our next issue.

Man's mind stretched to a new idea never goes back to its original dimensions
-Oliver Wendell Holmes

NINETEEN

Super Maximal Rep Training

In fitness, there's been a recurring theory floating around stating that performing high repetitions can dramatically increase a persons muscular definition. The premise of this theory is simply that performing high reps may cause the body to burn localized body-fat, thereby increasing the potential of getting ripped.

This getting ripped scenario happens, according to the theory, because after completing a certain number of reps, various fuel systems of a working muscle such as ATP and CP are depleted. The depletion of these fuels force the working muscle to begin using local deposits of fat as fuel making up for the energy deficit. Burning up stored body fat around a muscle would in turn, lead to an increase in definition. Not a bad theory, but does in work? To answer that question, lets explore where this theory originated.

Several years ago, there was an explosion of information on various methods of Eastern European strength and conditioning training for sports. In one particular method, an athlete would perform a series of extremely high repetitions of an exercise. The goal of this specific method was to increase an athletes muscle endurance level, as well as, increases their tolerance to pain induced by lactic acid build up. Eastern European sports scientists named this "Muscle Endurance" (ME) training.

ME training was extremely effective in increasing an athletes endurance, but there was one curious thing about the ME phase. It seemed that one of the by-products was a stark increase in an athletes muscular definition. The Eastern Europeans coaches didn't particularly care about their athletes getting ripped. Their focus was on improving athletic performance. So to them, this by-product was of little interest. It was only when western fitness experts began studying Eastern European methods that this discovered effect took on any importance.

Even with this information, the question is still, " Will high rep training actually work for the average person?" The answer in part is yes. Using super maximal repetitions can help increase muscle definition. This type of training may also increase muscle size in some individual who's muscle fiber type is such that they respond to super-maximal repetitions. Lets go over some previously un-mentioned realities of using this type of training.

First, lets establish just what super-maximal repetitions training actually means. To most people who exercise, high reps may mean between twenty-five or even thirty reps per set of an exercise. The fact is, twenty-five reps is not super- maximal. This number of reps will have little effect in getting you ripped.

According to Eastern European sports training doctrine, super-maximal reps may mean 100 or more reps per set. Not only are you performing 100 reps, but the exercise on a super-maximal repetition ME program are performed in a circuit manner, non-stop. This means several exercises are grouped together, and an athlete moves from one to another performing 100 reps per exercise. Two complete circuits are usually performed per work-out with up to twenty minute rest intervals between circuits.

If you do your addition correctly, this means that at the end of a muscle endurance workout, an athlete may have performed several hundred reps. Sounds pretty tough, doesn't it? Well it is. This level of intensity in using super-maximal repetitions training is an aspect many fitness people failed to understand when they talk about high rep training.

Another aspect of super-maximal repetition training, is that it takes months of training to build up the foundation necessary to withstand the demands of this method. Not just physically, but mentally as well. It's not a whole lot a fun performing a hundred or more reps, while at the same time, mentally focusing on dealing with the lactic acid burn within the muscle. You have to develop a strong self-discipline to complete the task ,as well as, the will to withstand the pain. But given time, the body will adapt to these demands.

Weight load selection is also a crucial aspect of using super-maximal repetitions. During this phase, weight loads should be between 30% to 50% of a persons one 1RM load. The percentages of weight loads are always calculated after a person takes a 1RM test, and testing is performed at the start of super-maximal repetition training.

To design a super-maximal repetition training program, you first must understand your own limitations, physically and mentally. If you're new to fitness, you may want to get some gym time in before you attempt this method. Also, if you find yourself easily board and like to change training programs frequently, you may also want to hold off on this type of training. On the other hand, if you're an individual who is experienced in fitness or sports and has the ability to mentally focus, this will be an excellent challenge for you.

To begin your own super-maximal repetition program, you first need to select the exercises. Keep the total number limited to around five to seven. Make sure you employ only the basic compound exercise such as; squats, bench press, leg curls, pulldowns, shoulder press, ab crunch, calf raise and so on. When you have selected your exercise, you'll then need to perform a one 1-RM on each exercise.

In order to safely work up to performing super-maximal repetitions, your program will need to be planned out for ten, twelve or even fifteen weeks, with two to three workouts per week. Starting out your first week, you should be using between 30 to 35 reps per set. From your calculations, make sure you use a weight load range that will allow you to complete a full set.

Since you'll be using light loads, do not let your ego get bruised or in the way. Remember it's more important to make the reps than it is using more weight. This is not a strength producing phase. If you can't make a set of thirty reps using 50% of your 1-RM, then drop the load down to 40% or 30%. Also, make sure you use the same amount of reps each workout for a complete week before you increase reps. Reps should be increased 5 to 10 reps per set each week depending upon your level of fitness.

As mentioned before, all the exercises are performed in a circuit manner one after the other. You'll need to take some time to adapt to this also. During the first week, take as long as you want in between each exercise. Allow yourself time to catch your breath before you begin the next one. When you're using a circuit method remember, always begin with the exercise that work the larger muscle groups, then work down to the smaller groups. When all your exercise are completed on the first circuit, take 10 to 15 minutes to re-group and begin the second set in a similar manner.

Over the weeks as you increase the reps, begin to perform two exercise non-stop then take your rest period. As the weeks go by, increase to three exercise before you take a rest period and so on. If your timing is right, your body will begin to adapt. So much so, that by the time you reach the last couple of weeks on your program, you'll be able to complete one whole circuit of exercise non-stop. At that point, take twenty minutes rest before you begin your second set. Remember, this is a very tough training program. Do not rush into it. Allow yourself plenty of time to adapt.

TWENTY

Will Power Training

The ability of an individual to achieve outstanding results even though their actions should, by all logic, dictate failure is one of life's great mysteries. This mystery is especially true in the arena of sports. There are those individuals who can train incorrectly and diet improperly, but on competition day, they are simply the best there is.

Luck? Born talent? A gift from above? Maybe. But a more acceptable answer may be found in an athlete's most powerful natural training aid - "willpower". Some individuals get results because their willpower wills them to. They have developed this power so strongly within themselves, that anything less than achieving complete victory is unacceptable to the very fabric of their being.

This optimal willpower development was never more apparent than in Arnold Schwarzenegger. A friend of Schwarzennegger's once said, "Arnold was not a genetically gifted bodybuilder and, compared to other bodybuilders of that time, he had many flaws in his physique. But, on the day of competition, Arnold was the best there was. He walked on stage and he owned it". Schwarzenegger had the ability to will himself to win.

The ability to focus your willpower is ultimately responsible for producing champions from the athletically and genetically un-gifted. It's also a lack of this willpower that can produce failures from the naturally talented, and cause other raising stars to flare, fade and fall.

Can anyone develop a willpower of granite? Many experts say yes. Developing your willpower is no different than developing any other talent. It takes time, practice, patience and a training plan. Willpower training begins with simply having a need which must be fulfilled.

The stronger the need, the stronger the willpower. It is important to understand that the need gives you the "why", and the why gives you the "way". If you do not have a why, you will not find the way.

The great motivational author Napoleon Hill often wrote, **"Anything the mind of a man can conceive and believe, the body can achieve."** Conceiving that "need" which must be believed and then achieved is always found first in a person's goals. You need to write down your goals and desires. If your goals are not written down they are not goals. They're just daydreams. Willpower development does not respond to daydreams. Many people will not write down their fitness goals because they do not want to take the chance of breaking a promise to themselves. Their internal dialogue goes something like, "If I write a goal down, I know I will not achieve it, so why lie to myself?" How can anyone develop the unstoppable will-power to overcome all obstacles with that kind of attitude?

For your willpower to respond to your goals, they must be written in great detail. The more detailed, the more likely you are to attain them. Write down exactly how much you are going to weigh, or how many inches you're going to gain, or what kind of shape you're going to be in on competition night. If your goals are vague, your willpower will be vague.

You must also state clearly when you plan to achieve your goals. Having a completion date for your goal helps the mind to fine-tune and strengthen the willpower. Not having an exact completion date weakens the willpower.

It is also very important not to plan conflicting goals. This causes many problems which eventually lead to an endless cycle of frustration. Conflicting goals are simply goals that negate each other and cause an inner "conflict". This inner conflict will usually manifest itself in some kind of self-sabotage or self-defeating actions. Do not write down goals such as; winning the nationals, raising a family, getting your master's degree and being the best salesman in your division all in the next six months. If you do you'll drive yourself (and all those around you) crazy. You must prioritize your goals in order for them not to conflict.

After you have written down your goals in exact detail, dated them and prioritized them to avoid conflict, you must examine why you want to attain your goals. It's not just having goals which develops the willpower. You have to know why you want them. Is it the goal itself you need to have, or is it the "things" the goal will bring you that are important? What is it? Recognition? Money? Self-confidence? It's okay to be honest with yourself on this one. The more honest you are in understanding why you want something, the stronger you'll develop the willpower to achieve it.

You also need to write down how you will feel and what will happen if you don't achieve your goals. This is a self-imposed peer pressure or guilt trip. Ask yourself, "What will I feel like if I do not achieve this goal? Think about what things not achieving your goals will take away from you. This part of willpower training hurts, because you must be brutally honest with yourself. Is this negative thinking? Not at all. If you know that failure will cause greater pain than doing the things you need to do to win, your willpower will respond by convincing you to do anything to avoid the pain of failure.

Lastly, developing willpower takes an unending flow of positive re-enforcement. You must surround yourself with positive influences and people. If you have negative people in your life, get rid of them. Remember, ultimately you will become like those with whom you associate. So take a good look around at the people you hang with. Most likely in a few years they'll be out of your life, but the effect they can have on you, either positive or negative may linger with you much, much longer.

TWENTY-ONE

The
Resistance
BALL

The resistance ball is a new workout device that can help you develop a tighter leaner and stronger body. It was introduced by Swiss physical therapists in 1965 as a physical conditioning device to help patients develop balance and maintain an increase in their reflex actions. Initially the ball was introduced in the United States by physical therapists and athletic trainers to supplement rehabilitation routines. Today, the body ball is being used extensively in group exercise classes, personal training sessions and at home. It is an inexpensive safe and effective way to tighten and tone your body especially your hips, abs, thighs and gluts. Plus it is a fun training device.

Resistance ball training incorporates your body weight to create resistance. The ball is unique in that it helps put your body in position you couldn't otherwise achieve. Exercises in this program are designed to create an overload with a minimum number of reps.

Proper form is essential. The key to proper form is good body position. Specifically, good position is one that precisely matches the motion of an exercise to the action of the muscle being targeted. There is only one body alignment for a given exercise that matches the force created by your muscles directly against the resistance. This means doing an exercise without deviating from the correct position. Each exercise in this workout is designed to match your movement to muscle action as closely as possible.

When working out with the resistance ball the correct sequencing of the exercises is important. By taking into consideration the various muscle roles as prime movers or synergistic in each exercise, you are able to vary the difficulty level of your routine. As a rule an exercise that isolates the prime mover should be performed just followed by an exercise that isolates the prime mover should be performed just followed by an exercise that stresses the synergetic role of muscles. For example glute bridges (isolation) should be performed first followed by wall squats (synergistic).

When working out with the resistance ball short rest intervals between sets and exercises is recommended. For best results, rest only 15 to 30 seconds between sets and 30 to 45 seconds between exercises. Table 1 and 3 show a resistance ball workout routines.

Although this workout is non impact and poses little risk of injury, it is still essential that you begin your workout with a five to ten minute warm up and end with a five to ten minute cool down. Warm up should be gradual, steadily increasing in effort until you begin sweating lightly. Reverse the procedure for your cool down.

Wall Squats: Strengthen quadriceps.
Muscles involved: Hamstrings and Gluteal muscles

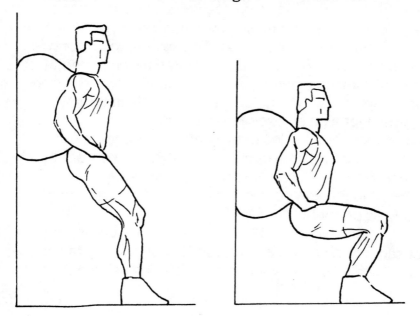

Stand with your back to the wall, adjust feet to shoulder distance, with toes pointing slightly outward. Place the ball in the
small of your back and lean against it, pressing the ball to the
wall. Lower yourself into a squatting position to a count of 2
seconds down and 4 seconds up. Descend until your thighs are
parallel to the floor.

One Legged Hack Squats
**Muscles Involved: Front of the thighs just above the knees,
as well as gluts and abs**

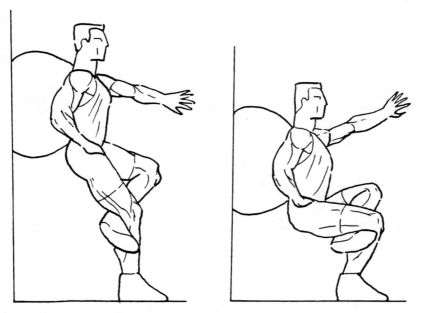

Place the leg to be worked under the center of your
body for balance. Place the other leg under the exercising leg.
Lower yourself until your thigh is parallel to the ground.
Focus on pushing off your heels. Exhale as you squat and
inhale as you come up.

Hamstring Bridges
Muscles involved: Strengthen your hamstrings

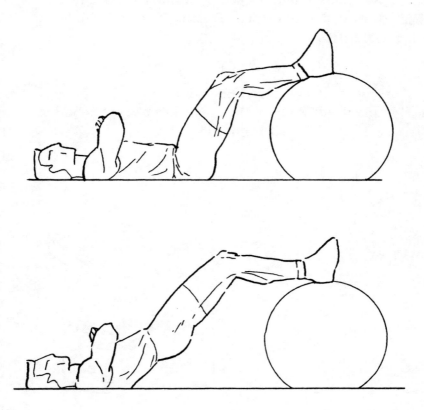

Lie on your back with your knees slightly bent and your heels and lower calves on the ball. Your head is on the floor with your hands on your abdomen. Raise your pelvis about 6 inches off the floor by squeezing your glutes together and by pressing your heels on the ball. Lower and repeat. Exhale as you press down, inhale as you lower your pelvis.

Dolphins
Muscles Involved: Strengthens spinal erectors, glutes and hamstrings.

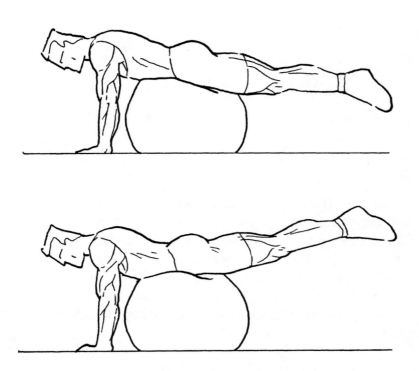

Kneel facing the ball. Lean forward until your pelvis is supported by the ball with your hands in front of the ball on the floor supporting your body. Position yourself on the ball to balance yourself. Feet should be together with your toes touching the floor. Raise your toes off the floor as high as possible. Keep your knees slightly bent. Lower your legs as close to the floor as possible and repeat.

Inner Thigh Raises
Muscles Involved: Strengthens leg adductors and inner thigh muscles.

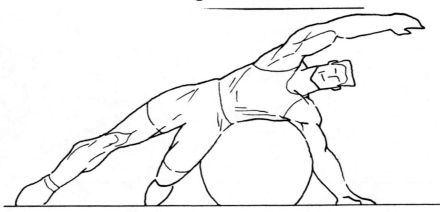

Lean sideways on the ball, placing it underneath your arm. Place your hand on the floor for balance. Your lower leg should be straight while your other leg is bent to help you maintain balance. Raise the foot of the lower leg about 12 inches off the floor, rotating your leg so that as you lift, your foot remains parallel to the floor. Do not touch the floor between repetitions. Exhale as you raise the leg and inhale as you lower it. Repeat on your other side.

Superman's / Muscles Involved: Strengthens back, glutes and leg muscles.

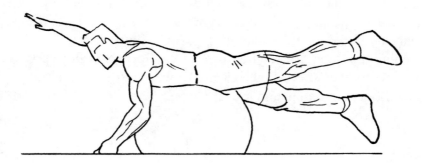

Spread your body over the ball at your midsection. Place your feet together with the balls of your toes touching the floor. Raise one arm and opposite leg together, keeping them straight allowing your back to extend and arch slightly. Gently alternate arms and legs with each repetition.

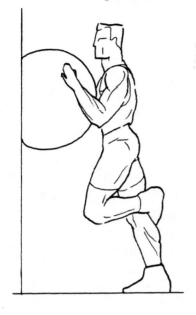

One Legged Calf Raises
Muscles Involved:
Strengthens calf muscles.

Stand facing wall, placing the ball between your chest and the wall. Lean forward and hold it in place. Place your hands on top of the ball for balance. Center your exercising leg below you for better balance and rest your other leg on the calf muscle of your exercising leg. Rise as high as possible on the ball of your foot, then slowly lower yourself until your heels touches the floor.

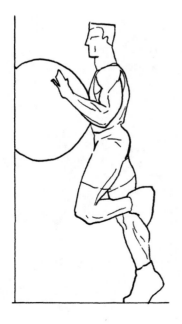

Back Extension
Muscles Involved: Strengthens the back and glute muscles

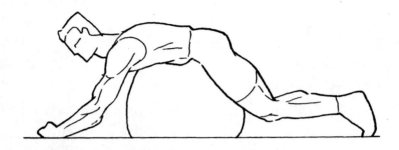

Spread you body over the ball so that it supports the midsection. Spread feet shoulder width apart. Place your hands behind your head and lower your body until your elbows touch the floor. Keep your back rounded with the curve of the ball. Raise your upper body one segment at a time. Raise your head and elbows then upper back and finally your lower back. Lower and repeat. Exhale as you raise your body and inhale as you lower it.

Crunches
Muscles Involved: Strengthens abdominal muscles.

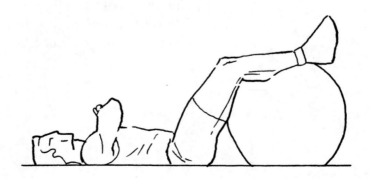

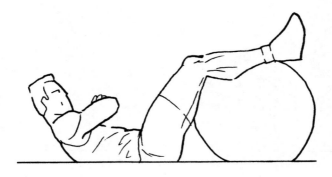

Lie on your back with your knees bent at 90 degree angle, heels resting on the ball. Place your hands behind your head to support your neck. Slowly raise your shoulders and upper back about 20 degrees off the floor. Hold it for one second than lower.

Push Ups
Muscles Involved: Strengthens chest, shoulders, and triceps muscles.

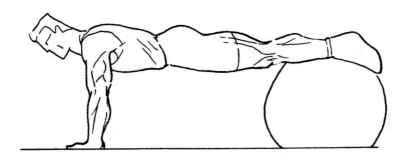

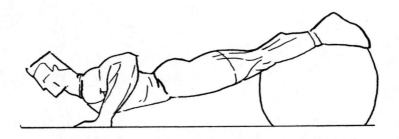

Spread out on the ball, face down position on the ball balancing on your shins and lower legs. Extend your arms placing your thumbs on the floor to shoulder distance apart to balance yourself. Lower yourself so your chest touches the floor. Push up to an extended position. Repeat. Exhale as you push up and inhale as you lower yourself.

Back Stretch
Muscles Involved: Stretches your spine, abs, and chest muscles.

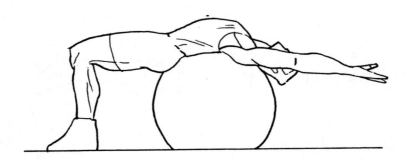

Lie backwards on the ball with your arms extended backwards. Keep your head on the ball. Knees bent at 90 degrees. Push with your feet, rolling yourself over the ball so that your arms and head move towards the floor. Reach with your arms. Hold for 10 seconds and repeat.

TABLE 1: Resistance Ball Routine I

Warm up   5 - 10 minutes

Exercises	Repetitions	Sets
a. Wall Squats	8-12	3
b. One Legged		
Hack Squats	6-10	2
c. Hamstring Bridges	7-11	2
e. Dolphins	8-12	1
f. Side Raises	15-20	2
g. One Legged		
Calf Raises	15-20	2
h. Supermans	10	1
i. Back Extension	10	1
j. Push Ups	15-20	3

Cool Down   5 - 10 minutes

Resistance balls come in various sizes. Your ball should be large enough so that when you sit on it, your knees bend at a 90 degree angle. A ball's diameter is measured in centimeters. A person 60 to 67 inches would probably use a ball 55cm; someone 68 inches or more would need one 65cm; and someone over 72 inches would use a ball 75cm. If in doubt, it is better to have a slightly larger ball than one that is too small. A ball should be inflated to the point where it still gives but is firm enough to roll. It will lose pressure and will need to be reinflated every three months.

In conclusion when working out with the resistance ball perform all exercises slowly and deliberately. Remember to follow the exercise descriptions carefully.

TWENTY-TWO

Elastic Resistance Training

Through proper instruction, Elastic Resistance can provide the means to safely improve muscular strength and endurance, range of motion, and flexibility. Also, it can easily fit in your gym bag and provide a fantastic workout. When using elastic tubing, to achieve gains in muscular strength, it is unnecessary to exercise at maximum levels. A tubing that produces 8 to 12 repetitions is equal to 70% to 80% of your maximum strength and is of a sufficient overload to produce strength gains. Twelve to 15 repetitions which is equal to 60 to 70% of maximum is recommended for beginners.

Elastic Resistance is perfect for the individual who wants to increase their knowledge base of resistance training for the: group fitness participant, personal training client, traveling or vacationing client, injured or rehabilitating client, athletes, youth and adolescent populations. This chapter will introduce you to every conceivable exercise for each region of the body. These exercises mimic every exercise that you can perform with free weights or machines. These exercises are highly effective and bomechanically safe.

General Guidelines

1. Select appropriate rubberized resistance based on your strength level. If moderate to maximal muscular fatigue isn't reached by your predetermined repetition goal, choose a heavier resistance. If unable to complete a minimum of 8 repetitions, choose a lighter resistance. Each exercise may require a different color or length or rubberized resistance.

2. Perform an equal number of repetitions with each arm or leg and work opposing muscle groups equally to avoid muscular imbalances.

3. Always control the resistance, especially during the return phase of the movement (3-4 seconds). You control the resistance tool, it doesn't control you.

4. Always inspect the rubberized resistance before each use for any nicks and tears that may arise from continued use. Avoid prolonged exposure to sunlight and salt or chlorine treated water.

5. Do not stretch rubber beyond 3 times its length.

6. Never tie two pieces of rubber together.

7. Perform each exercise as described.

8. When using a door strap or step strap, make sure it is secured prior to performing each exercise.

9. Consult your physician before beginning any type of exercise plan.

Elastic Resistance Stance Guidelines

Unless a specific foot position is noted when standing on tubing, follow this progression before moving to the next level of resistance.

Beginner: Place the middle of the tubing under the arch of front or rear of foot. Stand in a narrow staggered lunge stance.
Intermediate: Place the tubing evenly under the arch of both feet. Stand in a narrow square stance (feet hip width apart or slightly inside).
Advanced: Place the tubing evenly under the arches of both feet. Stand in a wide square stance (feet just outside hip width).

Elastic Resistance Body Alignment Guidelines

For exercises performed seated or standing:

1. Keep torso upright
2. Head and neck in neutral position
3. Shoulder square
4. Abdominals tightened to avoid excessive arch -ing of the back
5. Eyes focused straight ahead

Elastic Resistance Tubing Anchoring Guidelines

When anchoring the tubing, make sure it is securely attached to an outside object. Listed below are optional ways to anchor tubing

1. Around feet
2. Around door jam (door strap)
3. Around immovable objects ie: pole, weight machine, beam (double loop door strap).
4. Tubing nook ie: board with o-rings spaced every two inches (double loop door strap).
5. To step bench.

Before starting the exercise, move away from the tubing insertion to a point where the level of tension is constant throughout the entire range of motion. If the appropriate color tubing is chosen, there should be no excessive slack from the hand to the insertion.

REGION:CHEST

Seated Bent Arm Chest Fly (Pectorals)

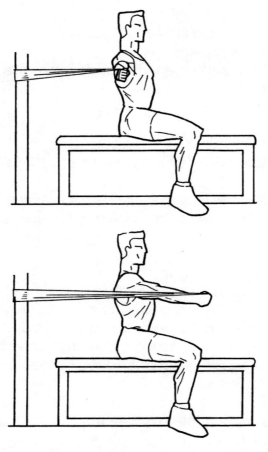

Sit on a bench with feet firmly on the floor of support position. Place tubing around a pole. Grasp the ends of the tubing with a regular grip. Start the motion with arms out to the side of the body. Keep elbows bent throughout entire exercise with wrists firm. Raise arms up and together. Squeeze pectorals by touching palms together at mid-chest height. Return to starting position and repeat.

Seated Bench Press (Pectorals)

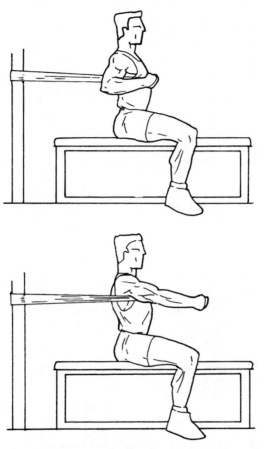

Sit on a bench with feet firmly on the floor of support position. Place tubing around a pole. Grasp the ends of the tubing with a regular grip. Start the motion with arms out to the side of the body. Extend the hands forward in a pressing motion until fully extended to mid-chest height. Return to starting position and repeat.

REGION: MID-BACK

Seated Row
Trapezius/Rhomboids/Latissimus Dorsi)

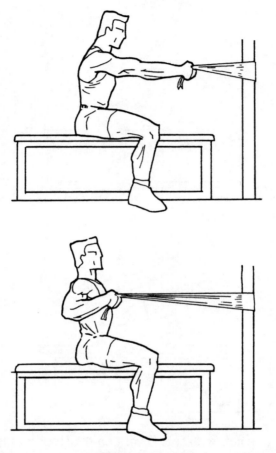

Sit on a bench with knees bent facing a post or pole. Place tubing around post. Grasp tubing and in a rowing motion pull ends towards you with elbows out. During the motion keep your back straight. Slowly extend tubing back to starting position and repeat.

Region: Anterior Upper Arm

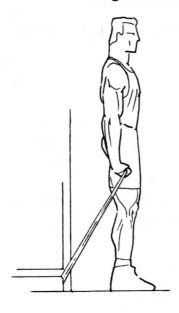

Standing Arm Curls
(Biceps)

Stand in a staggered position, narrow or wide stance. Place tubing under arch of front foot, or both feet, and soften knees. Grasp handles and straighten arms directly under shoulders with thumbs pointing forward. Bend elbows and progressively supinate forearms so palms face ceiling at hip level. Continue bending elbows until fists face ceiling. Palms of hands end facing front portion of shoulders with thumbs pointing out and away from sides of body. Finish with elbows directly under shoulders.

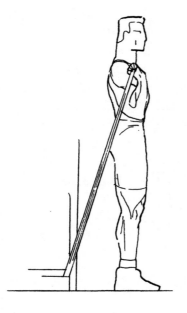

Region: Upper Leg

Seated Single Leg Press (Quadriceps/Hamstrings/Gluteals)

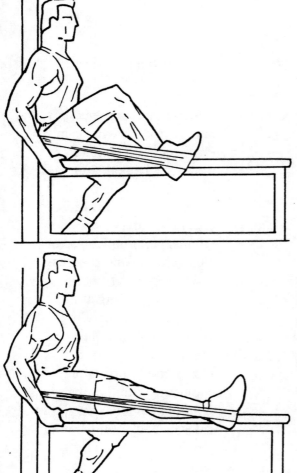

Start this exercise in a seated position on a low bench facing away from an extremely steady pole. Place the tubing twice around the post forming a strong loop. Place one foot against the end of the tubing with the other resting on the floor for support. While holding the sides of the bench strongly, press your leg forward until straight. Repeat motion with both sides.

Region: Posterior Upper Arm

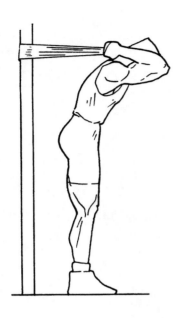

Standing Triceps Extension (Triceps)

Start this exercise by standing with your back towards a strong and sturdy pole. Wrap tubing around the pole and grab the ends behind your head. Your elbows should be pointing slightly higher than your shoulders. With your legs slightly bent, slowly extend your arms straight. Return to the starting position and repeat.

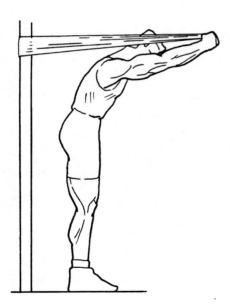

TWENTY-THREE

Speeding Up
Recovery

A person's inability to fully recover between workouts is one of the major "things that can go wrong" while on a fitness program. When incomplete recovery occurs, the body carries residual fatigue from the last training session into the next workout. Put a chain of these workout/incomplete recovery cycles together and the body will eventually become overtrained.

There are several post workout procedures a person can employ to help accelerate the body's natural recovery processes. These procedures aid in the removal of toxins and intercellular waste products which accumulate during a heavy training session. It's the build-up and retention of these naturally occurring cellular by-products that must be avoided if full recovery from training is to be attained. Remember that if the body fails to properly dispose of these by-products, they may linger causing internal malaise.

Procedures for speeding up the recovery process are usually grouped in two modified classifications. They are either active or passive. Active means they are performed at the end of a workout in some form of cool-down activity. Passive means they are performed during a rest period, away from the workout itself.

The first active procedure to begin the recovery process is to end every training session with an aerobic cool down period. Most individuals tend to just walk out of the gym following their last set. When this happens, toxins are allowed to pool in the body until some form of passive recovery is started. This is valuable recovery time being wasted. An aerobic cool down period begins the process of eliminating lactic acid from your system.

A well planned aerobic cool down period should last ten to fifteen minutes. Any aerobic activity will do. Stationary bike, treadmill or even a light jog are all excellent cool down activities. Keep the intensity light or moderate. If the cool down period is too intense, there will be no added recovery benefit. The best procedure to use to define what moderate is, is each individual's common sense and experience. Another active procedure to use during the cool down period is simple calisthenics movements such as shaking your arms out, light arm circles or swings, shoulder and hip rolls. These simple movements will also help to begin the recovery cycle. A period of light stretching performed at the end of the cool down is another important active procedure for the recovery process. You can use any stretching method you prefer.

A passive recovery technique which may be used is "hydrotherapy". Basically this means using water as a tool for speeding recovery. There are many forms of hydrotherapy. Hot whirlpool baths, Jacuzzi sport baths, sauna and steambaths all help to increase the body's ability to eliminate toxins while stimulating many internal systems which aid in recovery such as the endocrine system.

A hot shower is also an effective passive method to relax the muscles, stimulate the body's internal recovery systems as well as increasing blood circulation. Hot showers may be taken anytime, but they are particularly useful just before bed-time because they can induce deep sleep. A unique shower technique to increase circulation is to alternate hot and cold showers several times in a single session.

Another recovery tool is massage therapy. Massage after a workout helps to drain toxins and improves circulation. You do not always need a partner for a message. There are many self message techniques which can be easily be performed. Message therapy also speeds the recovery after a minor muscle or ligament tear or strain sustained from heavy training. It's these micro-traumas which cause both acute and chronic soreness. Both can be aided by massage by increasing the blood flow to the area.

To help increase the effectiveness of a massage, take a warm shower before the session and make sure to increase the room temperature to avoid chills. In local post workout message, use slow deep strokes working towards the heart to aid circulation.

Another great recovery aid is sleep. A physically active person must get a proper amount of sleep. The point is to get quality deep sleep. Stress, noise, too much partying and alcohol all can effect your quality of sleep. If you are training hard you should try to get a good solid eight hours. If your lifestyle permits, a half hour nap daily will also speed up recovery. It is important to go to sleep at the same time every night. When it comes to sleep, the body likes regularity.

Lastly, mental and emotional stress can hold back recovery and cause a person to fatigue and burnout just as easily as residual training stress. To help the body deal with this kind of stress, deep breathing exercises such as the kind used in yoga can help to relax the mind and de-stress the body.

Make the most of your recovery time. If you can incorporate a few of these techniques, you will not only speed up your recovery, you'll also get more out of your training.

Hot whirlpool baths, Jacuzzi sport baths, sauna and steambaths all help to increase the body's ability to eliminate toxins while stimulating many internal systems which aid in recovery such as the endocrine system

TWENTY-FOUR

Physical Detraining

It seems that in many aspects of life, its always easier to tear something down, than it is to build it up. This is especially true in fitness. Many of us know how difficult it is to create and maintain a pleasing physique. The dedication and self-discipline it takes to get your butt to the gym regularly, as well as, resisting some culinary delights to get ripped abs is something to be proud of. Unfortunately, many of us also know how easy it is to lose a pleasing physique. It may take months to show a noticeable increase in arm or chest size, but only a few weeks to notice a little extra size around the stomach if your training is interrupted. Sometimes, nature is cruel.

In fitness, the interruption of a persons regular training pattern is known as "detraining". Detraining comes in two forms, unplanned and planned. Unplanned detraining occurs because of a serious injury or illness. Planned detraining occurs because of a change in lifestyle, or takes place at the end of a competitive career, a competitive season or at the end of a yearly training cycle.

If for whatever reason detraining happens suddenly and unplanned, the effects, both physiological and psychological , are dramatic. Physiologically, negative detraining effects begin exceedingly quick. In less than two weeks after physical training stops, the body begins to show measurable declines in strength, metabolic rates and flexibility. After five weeks, it has been shown that in a trained athletes, metabolic rates such as cardiac output and cardio stroke volume can decrease as much as 19%

while the resting heart rate may increase as much as 6%.

Also during this period, one can expect to see a decrease in VO2 Max as much as 25%. One study even showed that the number of capillaries within a trained muscle may decrease up to 25% within three weeks of an interruption in training. The normal average is that an athlete will lose approximately 1% of their physiological functions per day during detraining.

Psychologically, abrupt detraining causes a host of problems at an even faster pace. These problems range from, loss of appetite, exhaustion, constant fatigue, headaches and sleep disturbances. The most serious of these functional problems is detraining depression. Detraining depression can be extremely debilitating, and in some cases, as serious as any other form of clinical depression.

In order to relieve the onset of negative side-effects from detraining caused by an illness of injury, an athlete may continue some limited training if possible. Obviously the extent of the injury or illness will determine this, along with a physicians recommendation. This limited amount of training which may be as little as two, ten minutes sessions per week , will help the athlete maintain some degree of physical readiness. These training sessions will decrease the severity of detraining side effects, especially depression.

Once the illness or injury is over, the rate of retraining should be aggressive. At this point, it is best advised that an athlete progress in training sessions from three 30 minute sessions per week, to four to five 60 minute sessions per week over a 30 day period. Training levels during this time should be between 50% to 60 % of the training levels prior to injury or illness.

If a detraining interruption is planned far in advance, many if not all the negative side-effects are avoided. Planned detraining periods are used to give an athlete a recovery period from training.

Many East European strength coaches plan out the detraining of the athletes well in advance of a detraining period. In some cases if an athlete is about to retire from competition at the national or international level, it is not uncommon for a detraining program to last three years. Many former East German Olympic athletes who retired after their last competition had planned detraining programs that lasted four to five years. For the average athlete who wishes to take a break from training, the detraining program should be planned for one to three months.

During this time, the object will be to decrease training time and intensity in a controlled manner. Many people tend to just stop training and not go to the gym. We know what happens when this occurs. If an athletes normal training pattern is three 90 minutes training sessions per week, this should be reduced down to two sessions of 30 minutes twice a week during a detraining period.

After this, a period of active rest may be used lasting two to four weeks. Active rest is basically physical activity not related to a persons normal training. If you're using progressive resistance weight lifting normally, your active rest period could include activities such as swimming, volleyball, tennis or golf.

At the end of an active rest period, an athlete may take one week of complete rest before a new training cycle begins. Complete rest is basically no physical activity whatsoever. This is the time when an athlete should sit down and plan out the next 12 months training cycle or competitive season. This new training plan should include one or even two other detraining periods.

.....In the world of the future, the new illiterate will be the person who has not learned how to learn.
                                                           Alvin Toffler

REVIEW QUESTIONS

A. Give several examples on how a person can speed up recovery in between workouts.

_____
_____
_____
_____
_____
_____
_____
_____
_____

B. Explain Muscle Endurance training.

_____
_____
_____
_____
_____
_____
_____
_____

C. What does it mean to have conflicting goals in fitness?

_____
_____
_____
_____
_____
_____
_____
_____

D. Explain the difference in weight load percentages between cycling phases of Activation, Strength and Muscle Hypertrophy.

_____
_____
_____
_____
_____
_____
_____
_____
_____
_____

E. Write the weight load percentages for a beginner strength phase.

_____
_____
_____
_____
_____
_____
_____
_____
_____

F. What does Detraining mean?

_____
_____
_____
_____
_____
_____
_____
_____
_____

TWENTY-FIVE

Exercise Description

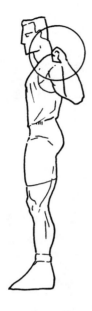

Region: Upper Leg

Squats

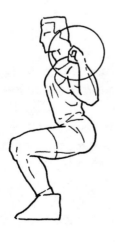

Stand in a wide stance with your feet slightly turning out while holding the bar on the back area of your shoulders. Keeping the head up and the back straight, bend your knees and lower yourself into a full squat position. Exhale as you raise back up to the starting position and repeat. Make sure you do not bounce at the bottom of the movement. Keep the complete motion under control.

Region: Upper Leg

Leg Press

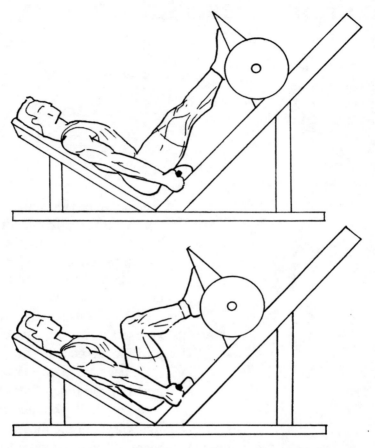

To properly perform this exercise, sit in the leg press machine and place your feet on the foot support. Make sure your feet are wider than shoulder width and are slightly turned out. Once you're in the correct position, push the weight load up and turn the support pins out. Lower the weight platform in a smooth controlled manner until the top of your thighs are parallel to the foot support and begin your repetitions. As you perform the leg press exercise, try not to bounce the weight load at the bottom of the movement.

Region: Upper Leg

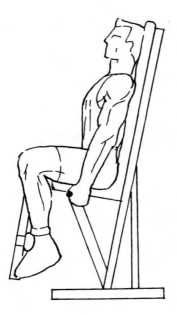

Leg Extension

To perform the leg extension correctly, sit in the leg extension machine with your knees pointing straight ahead and lined up with the joint on the machine. There is also a padded bar which moves the weight load; this bar should rest against the lower back of your shin, just above your sneaker top. When you are ready to begin the leg extension, simply raise the padded bar to a full extension,and return it to the starting position and continue your repetitions. Perform this exercise in a smooth and fluid motion.

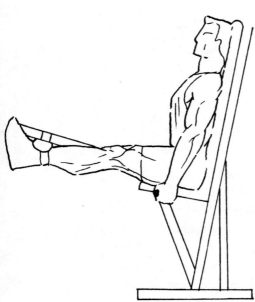

Region: Hamstrings

Leg Curls

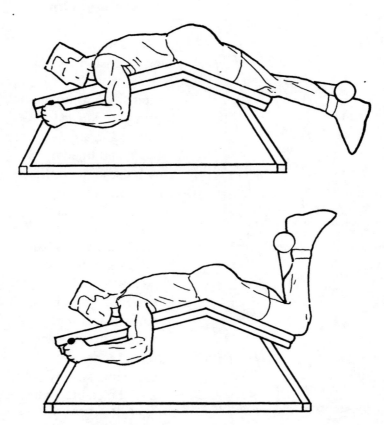

      To perform the leg curl exercise correctly, lay on the leg curl machine with your feet under the padded weight support. This bar should rest comfortably on the rear of your lower leg just above the top of your sneaker. If at all possible, use the kind of leg curl machine which has an arch. When you are ready to begin, simply raise the weight support towards your rear end and then return to the starting position. Make sure you raise and lower the weight in a controlled manner and use a comfortable full range of motion. Do not bounce the weight support off your rear end.

Region: Calves

Standing One Leg Calf Raise

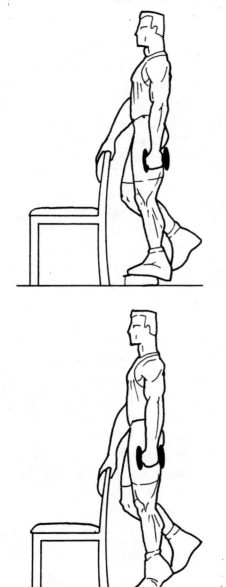

To begin this exercise, place the ball of your foot on a support several inches high. Hold a chair for balance in one hand as you hold a dumbbell in the other. Begin the movement by lowering your heel as far as your range of motion will allow. When they reach the bottom of the motion, raise up on the ball of your foot. The only moving joint will be your ankle, your knee, once in the correct position, does not bend during the movement. After your last rep, switch to other side.

REGION: UPPER BACK

Lat Pulldowns

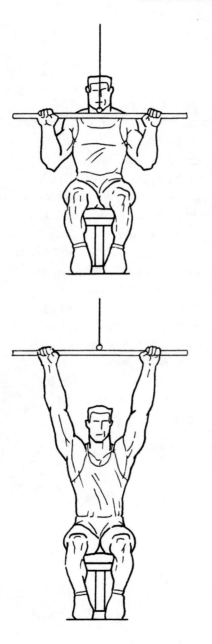

For this back exercise, use a lat pulldown machine or any overhead cable attachment. Using a straight bar, sit under the support pads and grasp the bar with a regular grip about shoulder width. When you are ready, pull the bar down to the top of your upper chest. Try not to go below the middle line of your chest. Touch the bar on your chest and begin your reps. When you're doing this type of pulldown, try not to lean back to far. Focus on keeping your back as straight as possible during the exercise.

REGION: MID-BACK

Seated Row

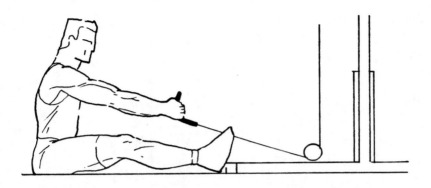

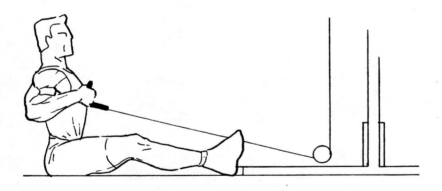

For this exercise, use the seated cable row machine or lower cable attachment. For the handle, use a regular t-bar. Grasp the handle and keep your knees slightly bent for stability. Begin the motion by pulling the bar towards your upper abdominals, keep you elbows out to the side as you pull. Do not rock and use your lower back, but instead try to keep the motion isolated on your back as you pull your elbows out and back as far a possible. When the bar touches the upper abs, control the movement back to the starting position.

REGION : CHEST

Bench Press

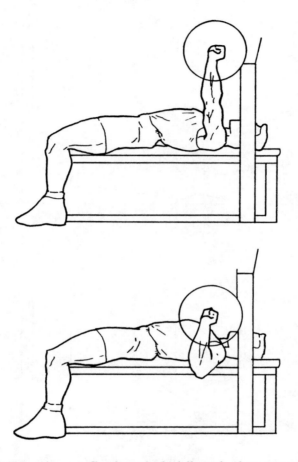

Lie back on a flat bench, holding the bar over the chest in a wide, overhand grip. Keeping the back flat and the feet stable, inhale as you lower the bar under control until it touches the chest at the nipple line. Push the bar back up explosively while exhaling and repeat.

REGION : CHEST

Pec Dec

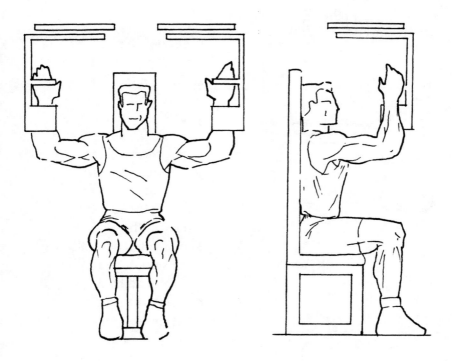

Sit on the Pec Dec machine with your arms out to the side. Place your forearms against the pads. Start the exercise by brining the pads together as you squeeze your chest. Do not push the pads with your hands, make sure you use just your forearms. Return to the starting position and repeat.

REGION : DELTOIDS

Shoulder Press

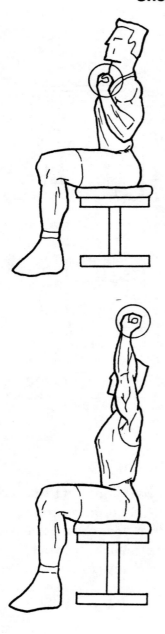

Sit on a bench and keep your feet solidly on the floor to give stability to your body. Rest the bar across your upper chest. When you're ready, begin the exercise by pushing the bar up over your head. When you reach full extension, lower the weight load back down to the starting position. As you're performing this exercise, try not to arch your back or move around as you lift the weight load.

REGION : DELTOIDS

Upright Row

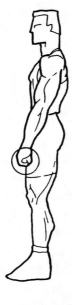

To perform this exercise, stand erect holding a barbell. When you're ready, begin the exercise by pulling the bar towards your chin. Make sure your elbows are high slightly above your shoulders. When you reach full motion, lower the weight load back down to the starting position.

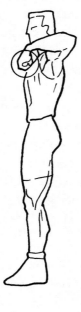

REGION : TRICEPS

Tricep Extension

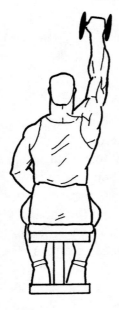

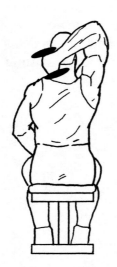

Sit on a bench and keep your feet solidly on the floor to give stability to your body. While holding a dumbbell in one hand, raise it above your head to the starting position. Begin the exercise by lowering the dumbbell behind your head. As you lower the weight, make sure your working elbow is held steady and pointed up. When you reach full motion behind your head, raise the weight load back down to the starting position.

REGION : BICEPS

Bicep Curl

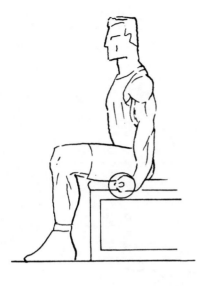

To perform this bicep exercise, hold a pair of dumbbells in your hands as you sit on the edge of a bench.. Your elbows will be in against your sides. Curl the dumbbells up towards your shoulders. As you do, try not to let your elbows move. Also, for safety sake, it's important that you do not swing the weight up. Use a concentrated effort to curl the weight in a controlled manner, and then lower it back down to the starting position. At this point repeat.

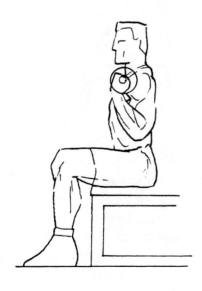

REGION : ABDOMINALS

Ab Crunch

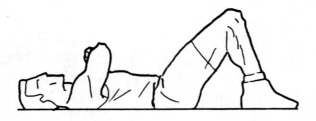

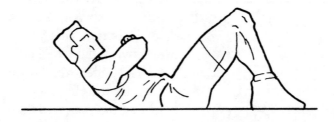

Start the ab crunch exercise by lying down on the floor with your legs bent at about a forty-five degree angle. Your hands should be folded across your chest. Start the crunch motion by bringing your shoulders off the floor in a circular motion as if you were going to roll into a ball. Make sure you keep your lower back against the floor during the whole crunch motion. When you reach your full range of motion, return to the start position and pause for a moment. This will help eliminate any momentum.

REGION : ABDOMINALS

Sit-Up

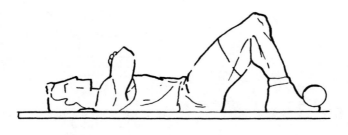

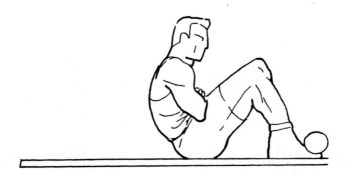

Start by laying down on the floor with your legs bent at slightly lower than a forty-five degree angle and your shoulders down as far as possible. Your hands can either be behind your head or folded on your chest. Once you're ready, start by bringing your shoulders off the floor in a downward circular crunch motion. As you progress through the crunch bend at your waist allowing the lower back to leave the ground. Come up until arms and chest are against your leg and return to the starting position. Try not to come off the floor as stiff as a board, but allow your back to roll up.

REGION : ABDOMINALS / OBLIQUES

Sit-Up Twist

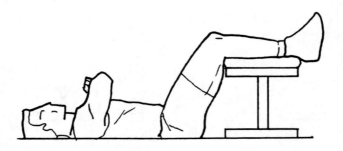

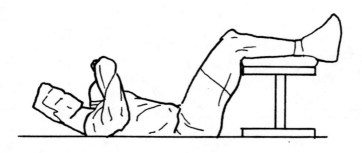

Perform this exercise in the same position as you did
for the ab crunch. This time instead of crunching straight up,
you're going to add a twisting motion as you crunch. Try to
bring you shoulders towards the midline of you body while
you keep your lower back on the floor. If your lower back
remains on the floor, the shoulders will stop the movement
before they reach the mid-line. This will assure that you do not
go too far and that you hit the proper range of motion.

BODY WEIGHT CALISTHENICS EXERCISES

Free Squat

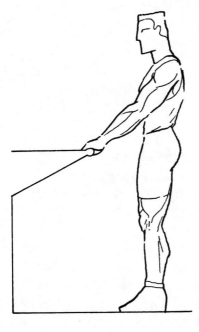

Stand in a wide stance with your feet slightly turning out while holding a support bar. Keeping the head up and the back straight, bend your knees and lower yourself into a full squat position. Exhale as you raise back up to the starting position and repeat. Make sure you do not bounce at the bottom of the movement. Keep the complete motion under control.

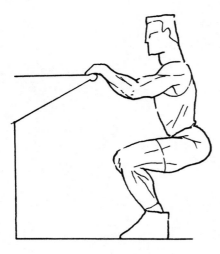

BODY WEIGHT CALISTHENICS EXERCISES

Pull Ups

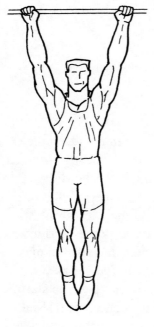

Start this exercise by hanging from the chin-up bar using a regular grip. Pull your body up until your chin is over the top of the bar, and slowly lower yourself back down into the starting position. Exhale as you pull you body up, and inhale as you lower yourself back to the starting position.

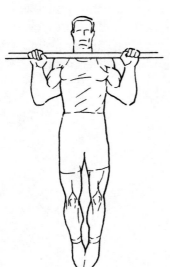

BODY WEIGHT CALISTHENICS EXERCISES

Chin Ups

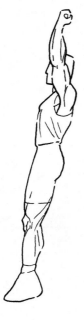

Start this exercise by hanging from the chin-up bar using a reverse grip. Pull your body up until your chin is over the top of the bar, and slowly lower yourself back down into the starting position. Exhale as you pull you body up, and inhale as you lower yourself back to the starting position.

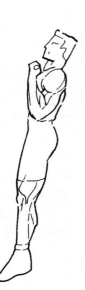

BODY WEIGHT CALISTHENICS EXERCISES

Push Ups

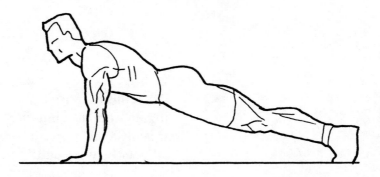

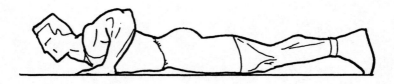

Start from a traditional pushup position. Keep your head up as you lower yourself to the floor until you chest touches the ground. Push yourself back up to the starting position as you exhale. Perform your pushups in three hand positions, close, shoulders width and wide.

FITNESS FOR THE NEW MILLENNIUM

Appendix I

Training Log

Fitness Personal Profile

Prior to beginning any physical exercise program, it is important that you consult with your physician on how this will impact your individual conditions. It is highly recommend that you see your physician before starting any fitness program.

NOTE: If you answer yes to any of the following questions, you must consult your physician and receive his/hers consent before beginning an exercise program.

Has your doctor ever said you have heart trouble?
Yes _____ No_____

Do you frequently have pains in your heart or chest?
Yes _____ No _____

Do you often feel faint or have severe dizziness?
Yes _____ No _____

Has a doctor ever said your blood pressure was high?
Yes _____ No _____

Has your doctor ever told you that you have a bone or joint problem such as arthritis that has been aggravated by exercise, or might be made worse with exercise?
Yes _____ No _____

Is there good physical reason not mentioned here why you should not follow an activity program if you want?
Yes _____ No _____

Are you over the age of 65 and not accustomed to a vigorous exercise?
Yes _____ No _____

How would you rate your present level of fitness on a scale from 1 to 10 (1 being unfit and 10 being the best shape you've ever been in). _____

Training Log Strength Test 1RM

NAME _____

STRENGTH TEST # _____

TESTING TIMES PER WEEK _____

Exercise:

(1)_____   Result _____
Set # 1 -Reps - Lbs   _____
Set # 2 -Reps - Lbs   _____
Set # 3 -Reps - Lbs   _____
Set # 4 -Reps - Lbs   _____
Set # 5 -Reps - Lbs   _____

Exercise:

(2)_____   Result _____
Set # 1 -Reps - Lbs   _____
Set # 2 -Reps - Lbs   _____
Set # 3 -Reps - Lbs   _____
Set # 4 -Reps - Lbs   _____
Set # 5 -Reps - Lbs   _____

Exercise:

(3)_____   Result _____
Set # 1 -Reps - Lbs   _____
Set # 2 -Reps - Lbs   _____
Set # 3 -Reps - Lbs   _____
Set # 4 -Reps - Lbs   _____
Set # 5 -Reps - Lbs   _____

Exercise:

(4)_____   Result _____
Set # 1 -Reps - Lbs   _____
Set # 2 -Reps - Lbs   _____
Set # 3 -Reps - Lbs   _____
Set # 4 -Reps - Lbs   _____
Set # 5 -Reps - Lbs   _____

Exercise:

(5)_____ Result _____

Set # 1 -Reps - Lbs   _____

Set # 2 -Reps - Lbs   _____

Set # 3 -Reps - Lbs   _____

Set # 4 -Reps - Lbs   _____

Set # 5 -Reps - Lbs   _____

Exercise:

(6)_____ Result _____

Set # 1 -Reps - Lbs   _____

Set # 2 -Reps - Lbs   _____

Set # 3 -Reps - Lbs   _____

Set # 4 -Reps - Lbs   _____

Set # 5 -Reps - Lbs   _____

Exercise:

(7)_____ Result _____

Set # 1 -Reps - Lbs   _____

Set # 2 -Reps - Lbs   _____

Set # 3 -Reps - Lbs   _____

Set # 4 -Reps - Lbs   _____

Set # 5 -Reps - Lbs   _____

Exercise:

(8)_____ Result _____

Set # 1 -Reps - Lbs   _____

Set # 2 -Reps - Lbs   _____

Set # 3 -Reps - Lbs   _____

Set # 4 -Reps - Lbs   _____

Set # 5 -Reps - Lbs   _____

Exercise:

(9)_____ Result _____

Set # 1 -Reps - Lbs   _____

Set # 2 -Reps - Lbs   _____

Set # 3 -Reps - Lbs   _____

Set # 4 -Reps - Lbs   _____
Set # 5 -Reps - Lbs   _____

Exercise:
(10)_____   Result _____
Set # 1 -Reps - Lbs   _____
Set # 2 -Reps - Lbs   _____
Set # 3 -Reps - Lbs   _____
Set # 4 -Reps - Lbs   _____
Set # 5 -Reps - Lbs   _____

Exercise:
(11)_____   Result _____
Set # 1 -Reps - Lbs   _____
Set # 2 -Reps - Lbs   _____
Set # 3 -Reps - Lbs   _____
Set # 4 -Reps - Lbs   _____
Set # 5 -Reps - Lbs   _____

Exercise:
(12)_____   Result _____
Set # 1 -Reps - Lbs   _____
Set # 2 -Reps - Lbs   _____
Set # 3 -Reps - Lbs   _____
Set # 4 -Reps - Lbs   _____
Set # 5 -Reps - Lbs   _____

Exercise:
(13)_____   Result _____
Set # 1 -Reps - Lbs   _____
Set # 2 -Reps - Lbs   _____
Set # 3 -Reps - Lbs   _____
Set # 4 -Reps - Lbs   _____
Set # 5 -Reps - Lbs   _____

Exercise:
(14)_____   test Result _____

Set # 1 -Reps - Lbs _____
Set # 2 -Reps - Lbs _____
Set # 3 -Reps - Lbs _____
Set # 4 -Reps - Lbs _____
Set # 5 -Reps - Lbs _____

Exercise:
(15)_____ Result _____
Set # 1 -Reps - Lbs _____
Set # 2 -Reps - Lbs _____
Set # 3 -Reps - Lbs _____
Set # 4 -Reps - Lbs _____
Set # 5 -Reps - Lbs _____

Exercise:
(16)_____ Result _____
Set # 1 -Reps - Lbs _____
Set # 2 -Reps - Lbs _____
Set # 3 -Reps - Lbs _____
Set # 4 -Reps - Lbs _____
Set # 5 -Reps - Lbs _____

Exercise:
(17)_____ Result _____
Set # 1 -Reps - Lbs _____
Set # 2 -Reps - Lbs _____
Set # 3 -Reps - Lbs _____
Set # 4 -Reps - Lbs _____
Set # 5 -Reps - Lbs _____

Exercise:
(18)_____ Result _____
Set # 1 -Reps - Lbs _____
Set # 2 -Reps - Lbs _____
Set # 3 -Reps - Lbs _____
Set # 4 -Reps - Lbs _____
Set # 5 -Reps - Lbs _____

TRAINING LOG
TIMES PER WEEK _____
REST INTERVALS (RI)_____
DATE START _____
ENDING_____

WEEK #   Workout #

1   date____   date____   date____
2   date____   date____   date____
3   date____   date____   date____
4   date____   date____   date____
5   date____   date____   date____
6   date____   date____   date____
7   date____   date____   date____
8   date____   date____   date____
9   date____   date____   date____
10   date____   date____   date____
11   date____   date____   date____
12   date____   date____   date____

WEEK 1

Exercise (1)_____

Set # 1 -Reps - Lbs   _____
Set # 2 -Reps - Lbs   _____
Set # 3 -Reps - Lbs   _____
Set # 4 -Reps - Lbs   _____
Set # 5 -Reps - Lbs   _____

Exercise (2)_____

Set # 1 -Reps - Lbs   _____
Set # 2 -Reps - Lbs   _____
Set # 3 -Reps - Lbs   _____
Set # 4 -Reps - Lbs   _____

Set # 5 -Reps - Lbs   _____

Exercise (3)_____

Set # 1 -Reps - Lbs   _____
Set # 2 -Reps - Lbs   _____
Set # 3 -Reps - Lbs   _____
Set # 4 -Reps - Lbs   _____
Set # 5 -Reps - Lbs   _____

Exercise 41)_____

Set # 1 -Reps - Lbs   _____
Set # 2 -Reps - Lbs   _____
Set # 3 -Reps - Lbs   _____
Set # 4 -Reps - Lbs   _____
Set # 5 -Reps - Lbs   _____

Exercise (5)_____

Set # 1 -Reps - Lbs   _____
Set # 2 -Reps - Lbs   _____
Set # 3 -Reps - Lbs   _____
Set # 4 -Reps - Lbs   _____
Set # 5 -Reps - Lbs   _____

Exercise (6)_____

Set # 1 -Reps - Lbs   _____
Set # 2 -Reps - Lbs   _____
Set # 3 -Reps - Lbs   _____
Set # 4 -Reps - Lbs   _____
Set # 5 -Reps - Lbs   _____

Exercise (7)_____

Set # 1 -Reps - Lbs   _____
Set # 2 -Reps - Lbs   _____
Set # 3 -Reps - Lbs   _____
Set # 4 -Reps - Lbs   _____
Set # 5 -Reps - Lbs   _____

Exercise (8)_____

Set # 1 -Reps - Lbs   _____
Set # 2 -Reps - Lbs   _____
Set # 3 -Reps - Lbs   _____
Set # 4 -Reps - Lbs   _____
Set # 5 -Reps - Lbs   _____

Exercise (9)_____

Set # 1 -Reps - Lbs   _____
Set # 2 -Reps - Lbs   _____
Set # 3 -Reps - Lbs   _____
Set # 4 -Reps - Lbs   _____
Set # 5 -Reps - Lbs   _____

Exercise (10)_____

Set # 1 -Reps - Lbs   _____
Set # 2 -Reps - Lbs   _____
Set # 3 -Reps - Lbs   _____
Set # 4 -Reps - Lbs   _____
Set # 5 -Reps - Lbs   _____

Exercise (11)_____

Set # 1 -Reps - Lbs   _____
Set # 2 -Reps - Lbs   _____
Set # 3 -Reps - Lbs   _____
Set # 4 -Reps - Lbs   _____
Set # 5 -Reps - Lbs   _____

Exercise (12)_____

Set # 1 -Reps - Lbs   _____
Set # 2 -Reps - Lbs   _____
Set # 3 -Reps - Lbs   _____
Set # 4 -Reps - Lbs   _____
Set # 5 -Reps - Lbs   _____

Exercise (13)_____

Set # 1 -Reps - Lbs   _____
Set # 2 -Reps - Lbs   _____
Set # 3 -Reps - Lbs   _____
Set # 4 -Reps - Lbs   _____
Set # 5 -Reps - Lbs   _____

Exercise (14)_____

Set # 1 -Reps - Lbs   _____
Set # 2 -Reps - Lbs   _____
Set # 3 -Reps - Lbs   _____
Set # 4 -Reps - Lbs   _____
Set # 5 -Reps - Lbs   _____

Exercise (15)_____

Set # 1 -Reps - Lbs   _____
Set # 2 -Reps - Lbs   _____
Set # 3 -Reps - Lbs   _____
Set # 4 -Reps - Lbs   _____
Set # 5 -Reps - Lbs   _____

WEEK 2

Exercise (1)_____

Set # 1 -Reps - Lbs   _____
Set # 2 -Reps - Lbs   _____
Set # 3 -Reps - Lbs   _____
Set # 4 -Reps - Lbs   _____
Set # 5 -Reps - Lbs   _____

Exercise (2)_____

Set # 1 -Reps - Lbs   _____
Set # 2 -Reps - Lbs   _____
Set # 3 -Reps - Lbs   _____
Set # 4 -Reps - Lbs   _____
Set # 5 -Reps - Lbs   _____

Exercise (3)_____

Set # 1 -Reps - Lbs   _____
Set # 2 -Reps - Lbs   _____
Set # 3 -Reps - Lbs   _____
Set # 4 -Reps - Lbs   _____
Set # 5 -Reps - Lbs   _____

Exercise (4)_____

Set # 1 -Reps - Lbs   _____
Set # 2 -Reps - Lbs   _____
Set # 3 -Reps - Lbs   _____
Set # 4 -Reps - Lbs   _____
Set # 5 -Reps - Lbs   _____

Exercise (5)_____

Set # 1 -Reps - Lbs   _____

Set # 2 -Reps - Lbs   _____
Set # 3 -Reps - Lbs   _____
Set # 4 -Reps - Lbs   _____
Set # 5 -Reps - Lbs   _____

Exercise (6)_____

Set # 1 -Reps - Lbs   _____
Set # 2 -Reps - Lbs   _____
Set # 3 -Reps - Lbs   _____
Set # 4 -Reps - Lbs   _____
Set # 5 -Reps - Lbs   _____

Exercise (7)_____

Set # 1 -Reps - Lbs   _____
Set # 2 -Reps - Lbs   _____
Set # 3 -Reps - Lbs   _____
Set # 4 -Reps - Lbs   _____
Set # 5 -Reps - Lbs   _____

Exercise (8)_____

Set # 1 -Reps - Lbs   _____
Set # 2 -Reps - Lbs   _____
Set # 3 -Reps - Lbs   _____
Set # 4 -Reps - Lbs   _____
Set # 5 -Reps - Lbs   _____

Exercise (9)_____

Set # 1 -Reps - Lbs   _____
Set # 2 -Reps - Lbs   _____
Set # 3 -Reps - Lbs   _____
Set # 4 -Reps - Lbs   _____
Set # 5 -Reps - Lbs   _____

Exercise (10)_____

Set # 1 -Reps - Lbs   _____
Set # 2 -Reps - Lbs   _____
Set # 3 -Reps - Lbs   _____
Set # 4 -Reps - Lbs   _____
Set # 5 -Reps - Lbs   _____

Exercise (11)_____

Set # 1 -Reps - Lbs   _____
Set # 2 -Reps - Lbs   _____
Set # 3 -Reps - Lbs   _____
Set # 4 -Reps - Lbs   _____
Set # 5 -Reps - Lbs   _____

Exercise (12)_____

Set # 1 -Reps - Lbs   _____
Set # 2 -Reps - Lbs   _____
Set # 3 -Reps - Lbs   _____
Set # 4 -Reps - Lbs   _____
Set # 5 -Reps - Lbs   _____

Exercise (13)_____

Set # 1 -Reps - Lbs   _____
Set # 2 -Reps - Lbs   _____
Set # 3 -Reps - Lbs   _____
Set # 4 -Reps - Lbs   _____
Set # 5 -Reps - Lbs   _____

Exercise (14)_____

Set # 1 -Reps - Lbs   _____
Set # 2 -Reps - Lbs   _____
Set # 3 -Reps - Lbs   _____

Set # 4 -Reps - Lbs   _____
Set # 5 -Reps - Lbs   _____

Exercise (15)_____

Set # 1 -Reps - Lbs   _____
Set # 2 -Reps - Lbs   _____
Set # 3 -Reps - Lbs   _____
Set # 4 -Reps - Lbs   _____
Set # 5 -Reps - Lbs   _____

WEEK 3
Exercise (1)_____

Set # 1 -Reps - Lbs   _____
Set # 2 -Reps - Lbs   _____
Set # 3 -Reps - Lbs   _____
Set # 4 -Reps - Lbs   _____
Set # 5 -Reps - Lbs   _____

Exercise (2)_____

Set # 1 -Reps - Lbs   _____
Set # 2 -Reps - Lbs   _____
Set # 3 -Reps - Lbs   _____
Set # 4 -Reps - Lbs   _____
Set # 5 -Reps - Lbs   _____

Exercise (3)_____

Set # 1 -Reps - Lbs   _____
Set # 2 -Reps - Lbs   _____
Set # 3 -Reps - Lbs   _____
Set # 4 -Reps - Lbs   _____
Set # 5 -Reps - Lbs   _____

Exercise (4)_____

Set # 1 -Reps - Lbs   _____
Set # 2 -Reps - Lbs   _____
Set # 3 -Reps - Lbs   _____
Set # 4 -Reps - Lbs   _____
Set # 5 -Reps - Lbs   _____

Exercise (5)_____

Set # 1 -Reps - Lbs   _____
Set # 2 -Reps - Lbs   _____
Set # 3 -Reps - Lbs   _____
Set # 4 -Reps - Lbs   _____
Set # 5 -Reps - Lbs   _____

Exercise (6)_____

Set # 1 -Reps - Lbs   _____
Set # 2 -Reps - Lbs   _____
Set # 3 -Reps - Lbs   _____
Set # 4 -Reps - Lbs   _____
Set # 5 -Reps - Lbs   _____

Exercise (7)_____

Set # 1 -Reps - Lbs   _____
Set # 2 -Reps - Lbs   _____
Set # 3 -Reps - Lbs   _____
Set # 4 -Reps - Lbs   _____
Set # 5 -Reps - Lbs   _____

Exercise (8)_____

Set # 1 -Reps - Lbs   _____
Set # 2 -Reps - Lbs   _____
Set # 3 -Reps - Lbs   _____
Set # 4 -Reps - Lbs   _____
Set # 5 -Reps - Lbs   _____

Exercise (9)_____

Set # 1 -Reps - Lbs   _____
Set # 2 -Reps - Lbs   _____
Set # 3 -Reps - Lbs   _____
Set # 4 -Reps - Lbs   _____
Set # 5 -Reps - Lbs   _____

Exercise (10)_____

Set # 1 -Reps - Lbs   _____
Set # 2 -Reps - Lbs   _____
Set # 3 -Reps - Lbs   _____
Set # 4 -Reps - Lbs   _____
Set # 5 -Reps - Lbs   _____

Exercise (11)_____

Set # 1 -Reps - Lbs   _____
Set # 2 -Reps - Lbs   _____
Set # 3 -Reps - Lbs   _____
Set # 4 -Reps - Lbs   _____
Set # 5 -Reps - Lbs   _____

Exercise (12)_____

Set # 1 -Reps - Lbs   _____
Set # 2 -Reps - Lbs   _____
Set # 3 -Reps - Lbs   _____
Set # 4 -Reps - Lbs   _____
Set # 5 -Reps - Lbs   _____

Exercise (13)_____

Set # 1 -Reps - Lbs   _____
Set # 2 -Reps - Lbs   _____
Set # 3 -Reps - Lbs   _____

Set # 4 -Reps - Lbs   _____
Set # 5 -Reps - Lbs   _____

Exercise (14)_____

Set # 1 -Reps - Lbs   _____
Set # 2 -Reps - Lbs   _____
Set # 3 -Reps - Lbs   _____
Set # 4 -Reps - Lbs   _____
Set # 5 -Reps - Lbs   _____

Exercise (15)_____

Set # 1 -Reps - Lbs   _____
Set # 2 -Reps - Lbs   _____
Set # 3 -Reps - Lbs   _____
Set # 4 -Reps - Lbs   _____
Set # 5 -Reps - Lbs   _____

WEEK 4

Exercise (1)_____

Set # 1 -Reps - Lbs   _____
Set # 2 -Reps - Lbs   _____
Set # 3 -Reps - Lbs   _____
Set # 4 -Reps - Lbs   _____
Set # 5 -Reps - Lbs   _____

Exercise (2)_____

Set # 1 -Reps - Lbs   _____
Set # 2 -Reps - Lbs   _____
Set # 3 -Reps - Lbs   _____
Set # 4 -Reps - Lbs   _____
Set # 5 -Reps - Lbs   _____

Exercise (3)_____

Set # 1 -Reps - Lbs   _____
Set # 2 -Reps - Lbs   _____
Set # 3 -Reps - Lbs   _____
Set # 4 -Reps - Lbs   _____
Set # 5 -Reps - Lbs   _____

Exercise (4)_____

Set # 1 -Reps - Lbs   _____
Set # 2 -Reps - Lbs   _____
Set # 3 -Reps - Lbs   _____
Set # 4 -Reps - Lbs   _____
Set # 5 -Reps - Lbs   _____

Exercise (5)_____

Set # 1 -Reps - Lbs   _____
Set # 2 -Reps - Lbs   _____
Set # 3 -Reps - Lbs   _____
Set # 4 -Reps - Lbs   _____
Set # 5 -Reps - Lbs   _____

Exercise (6)_____

Set # 1 -Reps - Lbs   _____
Set # 2 -Reps - Lbs   _____
Set # 3 -Reps - Lbs   _____
Set # 4 -Reps - Lbs   _____
Set # 5 -Reps - Lbs   _____

Exercise (7)_____

Set # 1 -Reps - Lbs   _____
Set # 2 -Reps - Lbs   _____

Set # 3 -Reps - Lbs   _____
Set # 4 -Reps - Lbs   _____
Set # 5 -Reps - Lbs   _____

Exercise (8)_____

Set # 1 -Reps - Lbs   _____
Set # 2 -Reps - Lbs   _____
Set # 3 -Reps - Lbs   _____
Set # 4 -Reps - Lbs   _____
Set # 5 -Reps - Lbs   _____

Exercise (9)_____

Set # 1 -Reps - Lbs   _____
Set # 2 -Reps - Lbs   _____
Set # 3 -Reps - Lbs   _____
Set # 4 -Reps - Lbs   _____
Set # 5 -Reps - Lbs   _____

Exercise (10)_____

Set # 1 -Reps - Lbs   _____
Set # 2 -Reps - Lbs   _____
Set # 3 -Reps - Lbs   _____
Set # 4 -Reps - Lbs   _____
Set # 5 -Reps - Lbs   _____

Exercise (11)_____

Set # 1 -Reps - Lbs   _____
Set # 2 -Reps - Lbs   _____
Set # 3 -Reps - Lbs   _____
Set # 4 -Reps - Lbs   _____
Set # 5 -Reps - Lbs   _____

Exercise (12)_____

Set # 1 -Reps - Lbs _____
Set # 2 -Reps - Lbs _____
Set # 3 -Reps - Lbs _____
Set # 4 -Reps - Lbs _____
Set # 5 -Reps - Lbs _____

Exercise (13)_____

Set # 1 -Reps - Lbs _____
Set # 2 -Reps - Lbs _____
Set # 3 -Reps - Lbs _____
Set # 4 -Reps - Lbs _____
Set # 5 -Reps - Lbs _____

Exercise (14)_____

Set # 1 -Reps - Lbs _____
Set # 2 -Reps - Lbs _____
Set # 3 -Reps - Lbs _____
Set # 4 -Reps - Lbs _____
Set # 5 -Reps - Lbs _____

Exercise (15)_____

Set # 1 -Reps - Lbs _____
Set # 2 -Reps - Lbs _____
Set # 3 -Reps - Lbs _____
Set # 4 -Reps - Lbs _____
Set # 5 -Reps - Lbs _____

AEROBIC TRAINING

Exercise: (1)_____ (2)_____

WEEK#	Date
1-2	_____
3-4	_____
5-6	_____
7-8	_____
9-10	_____
11-12	_____

Program # _____

Level	_____
Time / dis.	_____
Speed	_____

STRETCHING / FLEXIBILITY

Exercise:

(1)_____
(2)_____
(3)_____
(4)_____
(5)_____
(6)_____
(7)_____
(8)_____

WEEK#	Date
1-2	_____
3-4	_____
5-6	_____
7-8	_____
9-10	_____

Stretching Exercise (1)_____

Set # 1 - Reps =   _____
Set # 2 - Reps =   _____
Set # 3 - Reps =   _____
Set # 4 - Reps =   _____

Stretching Exercise (2)_____

Set # 1 - Reps =   _____
Set # 2 - Reps =   _____
Set # 3 - Reps =   _____
Set # 4 - Reps =   _____

Stretching Exercise (3)_____

Set # 1 - Reps =   _____
Set # 2 - Reps =   _____
Set # 3 - Reps =   _____
Set # 4 - Reps =   _____

Stretching Exercise (4)_____

Set # 1 - Reps =   _____
Set # 2 - Reps =   _____
Set # 3 - Reps =   _____
Set # 4 - Reps =   _____

Stretching Exercise (5)_____

Set # 1 - Reps =   _____
Set # 2 - Reps =   _____
Set # 3 - Reps =   _____
Set # 4 - Reps =   _____

Stretching Exercise (6)_____

Set # 1 - Reps =   _____
Set # 2 - Reps =   _____
Set # 3 - Reps =   _____
Set # 4 - Reps =   _____

Stretching Exercise (7)_____

Set # 1 - Reps =   _____
Set # 2 - Reps =   _____
Set # 3 - Reps =   _____
Set # 4 - Reps =   _____

Stretching Exercise (8)_____

Set # 1 - Reps =   _____
Set # 2 - Reps =   _____
Set # 3 - Reps =   _____
Set # 4 - Reps =   _____

Stretching Exercise (9)_____

Set # 1 - Reps =   _____
Set # 2 - Reps =   _____
Set # 3 - Reps =   _____
Set # 4 - Reps =   _____

Stretching Exercise (10)_____

Set # 1 - Reps =   _____
Set # 2 - Reps =   _____
Set # 3 - Reps =   _____
Set # 4 - Reps =   _____

TRAINING NOTES

Strength - Max. Tension a muscle can exert one time

Endurance - Amount of weight over Time 2 Reps min/Static

Hypertrophy - Mass based on Genetic/Sex/Workout/Substances

Power - Max. Force in a period of Time

Tone - Muscle firmness

Definition - outline of muscle groups (genet./Training/diet)

Plyometrics - Activities That Stretch muscle before contract

Progressive Overload - Gradual increase of load, causing
The Body To react To Adapt To increased load.
- Intensity
- Duration
- Frequency
- # of Exercises

(*) 48-72 Hours untill OVER COMPENSATION

(*) Must work muscle 2x per week

Min. Overload   2x week 1set x (8-12)reps @ 70-89% 1RM
                 8-12 exer.

Rest - Min. 1 minute Rest Between exercises

Work out = Warm up; Exercise; Cool down

(*) STEP LOADING - 2/3 weeks progressive Increase 1 week redu
        - Loading progression Blocks
        - Regeneration Blocks

(*) Phases
    4-12 weeks

(*) cycles of Training for specific goal

Strength	100-85 x	(1-7) x	(1-5)
Mass	80-70 x	(8-12) x	(1-5)
Endur.	50-70 x	(12x20) x	(1-5)
Defin.	30-50 x	(20-50) x	(1-5)